THE FOOD ALLERGY FIX

The

FOOD ALLERGY FIX

AN INTEGRATIVE AND EVIDENCE-BASED
APPROACH TO FOOD ALLERGEN DESENSITIZATION

SAKINA SHIKARI BAJOWALA, MD

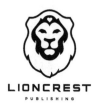

LIONCREST
PUBLISHING

THE FOOD ALLERGY FIX

An Integrative and Evidence-Based Approach
to Food Allergen Desensitization

ISBN   978-1-5445-1158-0 *Paperback*

       978-1-5445-1157-3 *Ebook*

To my parents, for raising their daughters to believe that changing the world was not only a possibility, but rather the expectation. All little girls should be so blessed with faith in their own promise.

To my husband, for being in equal measure my companion, compass, cheerleader, and drill sergeant. You believed I had a story worth telling. If not for you, this book would still be a collection of ideas in my head, rather than printed here on the page.

To my sons, for teaching me what it means to be fully invested in the fruits of my labor. In you, I see a better tomorrow. Being your mother is my greatest pride and deepest joy.

To my employees, for having faith in my vision of healthcare, and for treating our patients like family. Your compassion comes through in all you do.

And to my patients and their families, for their pioneering spirit and dedication to a safer world for all children with food allergies. You are some of the bravest people I will ever have the privilege to care for.

Thank you.

CONTENTS

INTRODUCTION

Attending a Chicago Cubs baseball game is a dream come true for a seven-year-old baseball fan living near the Windy City. But when you're a seven-year-old baseball fan with a *peanut allergy*, Wrigley Field isn't just the "Friendly Confines" in which to enjoy America's favorite pastime—it's also a potential minefield of dangerous peanut residue.

Charlie is that seven-year-old. He sits in front of me today, grinning from ear to ear because he knows he will soon be watching his beloved Cubbies *live in action*! He keeps wiggling while sitting on the exam table, unable to contain his excitement. Across the room, Charlie's mother rapidly taps her fingers together, her anticipation tempered by a twinge of anxiety. Today is Charlie's food allergen desensitization graduation, a milestone that's been in the works since he first stepped foot into my office more than a year ago.

Before he visited my clinic, Charlie had been rushed to the emergency room multiple times due to accidental peanut exposure. So it seems nothing short of a miracle that today, he will eat *twenty-four peanuts* in my office! How can this be? Well, Charlie has been pursuing a program of oral immunotherapy (OIT) to gradually increase his tolerance to peanuts. After today's medically supervised graduation is complete, he will be able to eat peanuts and walk confidently into "peanutty" situations instead of avoiding them entirely. This is no small feat, considering the restrictive lifestyle Charlie was leading before therapy.

Until he began treatment, Charlie's parents took a commonly advised approach to handling his peanut allergy: strict avoidance. Did it keep Charlie safe? Sure, but it also led to lifestyle limitations for both him and his family. There were school activities he could not participate in, places he could not go. Grocery shopping was ominous: would they miss something on a label? Birthday parties and eating out felt dangerous rather than fun. And a Cubs game? Out of the question. It was simply too anxiety-provoking.

The long road from avoidance to tolerance ends today! Charlie's exam room is filled with balloons and homemade signs, and my medical assistants poke their heads in the door as they walk past to offer their congratulations. In the corner sits a basket of peanut M&M'S and Reese's candies next to an *enormous* golden trophy in the shape of (you guessed it!) a peanut. To say Charlie and his family are ready for this day is an understatement—his freedom has been a long time coming, and they can taste it.

Charlie has now completed the entire peanut desensitization protocol. That's an incremental, highly precise, and medically supervised allergen-dosing process that can help patients better tolerate foods they are highly allergic to. Over the past year, Charlie and his family have been coming to my office every other week for *updosing*, a supervised increase in the amount of food allergen consumed. In Charlie's case, I administered doses of peanut protein. After each updose, Charlie was observed for an hour. Once it was clear he had fully tolerated the dose, I sent Charlie and his family home with detailed dosing instructions to follow until our next visit. This process continued throughout the year and brought us to this moment. Just think—a year ago, Charlie couldn't even consider eating a bakery cookie or going to many sporting events due to the risk of accidental peanut exposure. Today, on his peanut graduation day, he is going to eat two dozen whole peanuts—one full serving—right in front of me.

Charlie's parents and I watch as he eats peanut after

peanut successfully. Everyone in the room is ecstatic and smiling, but the biggest smile is reserved for Charlie's cherubic face. And why not? He knows that before he leaves my office, he will have earned his long-awaited Cubs day out. One hour after eating his twenty-fourth peanut, the room erupts in cheers! Charlie's entire family celebrates together and shares in the joy of the moment. This includes his younger sister and his little baby brother, who was born just a week after Charlie started his therapy.

Stories like Charlie's make me feel incredibly proud to be an allergist. In fact, graduations are my favorite days in the office. As soon as a child graduates, the halls are filled with cheers and laughter. This isn't just a celebration of the child who is graduating, though. It is also an echo of hope for those children who are present in the office that day for their initial consultations. Along with their families, they peek their heads out of their exam rooms when they hear the commotion, and the significance of what they are witnessing starts to set in. Suddenly, food allergy freedom feels like an accomplishable goal, not a long shot.

FILLING THE GAPS IN FOOD ALLERGY TREATMENT

I finished my fellowship in allergy and immunology in 2008, having been trained in all the standard diagnosis and management strategies for allergies. This included the process of desensitization, a precise method of safely introducing into the body substances to which a patient is allergic. We had desensitization protocols in place for environmental allergies such as pollen, dust mites, animals, and mold. We had desensitization strategies in place for antibiotics and even chemotherapy, but interestingly enough, not for food allergens. This always puzzled me because I believe food allergies are arguably more impactful to safety and quality of life than a drug allergy. They're certainly more dangerous than an environmental allergy, and we've been desensitizing for aeroallergens for more than a century.

For years, the only services my colleagues and I could offer patients with food allergies was to identify the allergen, prescribe emergency medication in case of accidental exposure, and advise strict food allergen avoidance. That was it. It felt stiflingly limiting because I knew we had the background knowledge needed to create desensitization protocols for foods. So what was stopping us from doing more? The truth was, we simply didn't have enough experience in performing food desensitization to tease out the nuances of the therapy and optimize it for patients.

I felt stuck. I was peddling fear instead of offering solutions that would inspire a better quality of life for the children who sat before me. "You're allergic to this food. It could kill you," was all I had to offer. "Don't ever eat it.

Stay away from it. A reaction could occur at any moment, so read the labels. Here's some injectable epinephrine. See me in a year." I was failing them, and I could feel it.

Then came the catalyst to change. During my allergy and immunology fellowship, my oldest son developed hives upon ingesting mixed nuts, and we discovered he had a hypersensitivity to peanut, cashew, and pistachio. We were prescribed an EpiPen and started avoiding these foods entirely, including items labeled for possible cross-contamination. Here I was, simultaneously living the life of an allergist and an allergy mom. My youngest son was born at the end of my fellowship, and he inexplicably began developing hives as I nursed him. I followed a short-term elimination diet and learned that highly acidic fruits were triggering his rash. Happily, my youngest was able to introduce citrus and berries within a few months, and my oldest outgrew his peanut and tree nut allergy at age four. This story is not typical: only 20 to 30 percent of young children with peanut allergies outgrow them spontaneously, and the other 70 to 80 percent will have their food allergies for life.

When my son outgrew his peanut and tree nut allergies, it quite literally changed our lives. I could distinctly see the difference in the quality of our life before and after resolution, and it was so freeing! I watched my son enjoy the same activities as his peers with no special restrictions, no emergency medication waiting in the wings. And I no longer had to question my family over every dish during the holidays with my broken record of "Stop! What's in that?"

I wanted every food allergy family to experience the freedom mine had been blessed with. So I began exploring desensitization options. I researched ways to transition what allergists and immunologists *already* knew about treating environmental and drug allergies and apply it to the management of food allergies. Although my colleagues and I had long recognized the gaps in our abilities to offer food allergy patients actual solutions to their problems, my own personal experience lit a fire inside me. I knew it wasn't enough for me to turn to one more child and say, "I'm sorry I have to give you this news, but you have a food allergy." I hated watching their eyes tear up, a sense of helplessness overtaking the room. That all ended in 2011 when I began performing food allergen desensitization. I still make people cry every day, but now, they're tears of joy.

"There's never been a more exciting time to have this food allergy," I tell the children in my office, "because we have real treatment options now. Together, we're going to make you better."

THE FOOD ALLERGY PROBLEM

The title of this book is *The Food Allergy Fix*, but before we can dive into the solution, we must first examine what's broken. So what is an allergy? Simply put, an allergy is an overreaction on the part of the immune system to a foreign substance that should, under normal circumstances, be well tolerated. Reactions can cause symptoms ranging from a mildly itchy mouth to a rapidly progressive, multisystem reaction known as anaphylaxis, a condition that can be life-threatening.

I firmly believe there is an epidemic of food allergies in the modern world. In any given classroom in the United States, two children will have a potentially life-threatening food allergy, a significant issue from both a safety and a health-care utilization/cost perspective. In fact, the economic cost of food allergies is a staggering $25 billion per year.[1]

About 3.6 percent of the US population has a food allergy, as do 8 percent of children. Of these kids with food allergy, 38.7 percent experience severe reactions to their allergens, and 30.4 percent have more than one allergy. The most common food allergens include peanuts and tree nuts (almonds, hazelnuts, cashews, pistachios, walnuts, pecans,

---

[1]   R. Gupta, D. Holdford, L. Bilaver, A. Dyer, J. L. Holl, and D. Meltzer, "The Economic Impact of Childhood Food Allergy in the United States," *JAMA Pediatrics*, November 2013, https://www.ncbi.nlm.nih.gov/pubmed/24042236.

Brazil nuts, and macadamia nuts), milk, eggs, soy, wheat, fish, shellfish, and seeds.[2]

What's the deeper meaning behind these statistics? The food allergy problem goes beyond the numbers, impacting children and their families who feel hopeless and caged in by an allergy diagnosis. This needn't be the case. In this book, I hope to present a practical alternative to the de facto strategy of strict avoidance and to propel my colleagues who are board-certified in allergy and immunology to employ desensitization to help better serve our food-allergic patients. We already have the background knowledge and the skillset, but we need some forward motion!

There is a steadily growing community of board-certified allergists offering food allergen desensitization therapy to their patients, and I am proud to be a member and contributor. In this book, I aim to share my own experiences and give patients and families the medical background they need to discuss treatment options for food allergy with their own doctors. I also hope to inspire my colleagues who are intrigued by the concept of doing more for our patients but are feeling restrained somehow due to a lack of institutional support, information, or even cheerleading. I want to help them realize they also have

---

2   "Food Allergy Facts and Statistics for the U.S." https://www.foodallergy.org/sites/default/files/migrated-files/file/Final-FARE-Food-Allergy-Facts_statistics.pdf.

the ability to bring this potentially lifesaving therapy to their patients in such a way that makes a widespread, meaningful impact on the treatment of the disorder. As Ralph Waldo Emerson said, "Do not go where the path may lead, go instead where there is no path and leave a trail." It's time for us to forge the trail.

WHY SHOULD YOU READ THIS BOOK?

Another one of my goals in writing *The Food Allergy Fix* is to reveal to families of children with food allergies that another world exists, a world where food allergies don't hold your child and your family back. I will give you the tools you need to be proactive and help take control of the food allergy rather than the other way around. I will educate you on how the immune system works and offer tips and tricks to reduce body-wide allergic inflammation. I will also discuss food allergen OIT as a potentially life-changing therapy. What can you get out of it all? The treatment that might propel your family from being held captive by food allergy to living freely.

That's what I *will* do, but what about what I *won't* do? First of all, I will not judge you for your choices. If your child and your family decide you'd like to continue with strict avoidance after reading this book, I support you. I am confident in the knowledge that you at least now know an alternative management strategy for food allergy exists. I couldn't live with myself if I didn't shout the benefits of OIT from the rooftops, because I believe it can save lives. However, my intention is only to share information, never to judge or discredit the path you choose to take for your family.

Second, while I will offer an overview of food allergen desensitization in the pages of this book, this is absolutely *not* a do-it-yourself manual. **OIT must be done under the medical supervision of a board-certified allergist.** *I repeat*: **Do not attempt any of the techniques described in this book at home! It could be fatal.**

I know on its face, desensitization seems intuitive. It's not rocket science, and I won't pretend it is. The difficulty lies not in the theory behind the science or in the development of a protocol but rather in its safe, practical implementation. I obsessively tune in to each detail for my patients, ensuring there are no dosing mistakes. I have learned to recognize when the right time is to dose and when to wait. I know when to reduce a dose, when to add adjunctive medications or supportive therapies, and how to handle and adjust for allergic reactions during the process. As a board-certified allergist and immunologist with nine years of postgraduate medical education and over a decade of hands-on clinical experience, it is my job to know these things. But as a parent, regardless of how well you know your own child, you will not have the medical experience necessary to supervise this process yourself. Bottom line? *Don't* try this at home. Get it? Got it! Good.

Now that we're clear, let's discuss the science and history of allergen desensitization—and how it can change the lives of food allergy patients around the world.

PART ONE

THE BACKGROUND: FOOD ALLERGIES AND DESENSITIZATION

CHAPTER ONE

WHY DO FOOD ALLERGIES DEVELOP?

Sophia, a bubbly six-month-old with wispy curls on top of her head, sits on her mother's lap and curiously reaches for my stethoscope as I examine her. As her parents recount her story, I learn that Sophia developed eczema three months ago. Her mother took Sophia to a dermatologist, who appropriately advised both a topical steroid ointment and a moisturizer to treat the rash. Although standard in the management of eczema, neither of these measures was helping Sophia's rash. To test for possible food allergies, Sophia's primary care pediatrician suggested Sophia's mother attempt a short-term elimination diet while breastfeeding. After eliminating milk, eggs, soy, and nuts from her own diet, Mom noted that Sophia's eczema improved. The pediatrician had encouraged Sophia's mother to slowly reintroduce the eliminated foods back into her diet, but Mom was worried about triggering a flare-up of the rash. She continued her own elimination diet and figured she could add the foods back once Sophia was older and was eating solid foods herself. It was hard work to maintain the diet, but Mom saw that elimination was working to keep Sophia's skin clear, and she wanted to do what was best for her baby.

At a family party last month, her parents explain, a well-meaning relative offered Sophia a bite of a muffin which contained baked egg. When their sweet little girl immediately developed itchy hives around her mouth, they knew it was true: Sophia had food allergies. They had their first clues when Sophia's eczema improved after her mother's dietary elimination. Now, the more acute presentation of hives removed all doubt. She had been doing so well, and now this! Sophia's parents were devastated.

THE ALLERGIC MARCH

Sophia's symptoms illustrate the typical progression of the *allergic march*, a progressive constellation of atopic (allergic) disorders that present in early childhood. In classic presentations, the first symptom to appear is eczema, an itchy skin rash that commonly appears on the cheeks,

extremities, and skin folds. Children may simultaneously exhibit signs of food hypersensitivity such as hives,
swelling, vomiting, diarrhea, or respiratory reactions. The
next disorder to present is commonly allergic rhinoconjunctivitis triggered by environmental allergens (pollens,
mold, animals, dust mites, etc.). It is hallmarked by nasal
congestion, runny nose, sneezing, and itchy eyes. Finally,
the child may begin wheezing and coughing periodically,
leading to an eventual diagnosis of asthma. This is not
to say that every child who has eczema, food allergies,
environmental allergies, or asthma will develop all four
conditions. We do know, however, that the allergic march
is a well-defined group of related atopic disorders that
tend to cluster together.

Most of the time, the allergic march starts in infancy, but
exactly how this process is triggered is not completely
understood. There is certainly a genetic component,
as atopic conditions are commonly shared among rel-
atives. However, the genetic propensity to develop allergic
disease is only one part of the picture. We know that genetically identical twins raised in different environments may
go on to express different health conditions. Why might
only one of a set of identical twin siblings develop allergies
or asthma while the other is spared? The answer lies in
epigenetics. Epigenetics is the study of heritable changes
in gene expression. Here, there's no altering of the DNA
sequence, just the activation of that gene. It's analogous

to a light switch being flipped on or off. You always have the wiring, the filament, and the bulb. However, the light only shines when the switch is flipped, sending electricity to power the existing hardware. What happens when only one twin develops allergies? Certain environmental exposures have activated those gene sequences. In other words, one twin's switch got flipped.

Any discussion of epigenetics in allergy raises an important question: Exactly which environmental factors trigger the expression or nonexpression of a genetic predisposition for allergic disease? Although the allergic march typically begins in infancy, the march may, on occasion, start later in childhood following an immune-stimulating event, such as a significant viral illness. I typically advise against introducing new foods during or immediately following significant infections for this very reason. Similarly, routine pediatric vaccinations, by design, stimulate a protective immune response to dangerous pathogens. Having personally witnessed tragic outcomes from vaccine-preventable illnesses, I enthusiastically encourage all my patients to be fully vaccinated. However, I do err on the side of caution and advise families of young children to wait one full week after vaccination before introducing new foods into a child's diet. The aim is to limit introduction of potential allergens when the switch might be temporarily stuck in the on position.

NATURE VERSUS NURTURE: ALLERGIC MARCH EDITION

Nature versus nurture has long been debated in psychology, but there's not much debate in the world of immunology: as mentioned above, *both* contribute to the progression of the allergic march. We already know that our genetic code lays the framework for susceptibility to allergy. Let's now discuss some epigenetic factors impacting the expression of allergic disease. Consider, for example, the hygiene hypothesis—a theory that states the oversanitization of our environment can interfere with the normal development of the immune system. Our immune systems are evolutionarily designed to have exposure to various microbes early in life as part of the normal training and development of the immune system. When we don't see these organisms in infancy and early childhood, it affects the gut biome, which is the population of gut flora (microorganisms) in your gastrointestinal (GI) tract. This "dysbiosis" can ultimately interfere with the proper training of the immune system and predispose to the development of allergy.

As an example of environmental influence on GI flora, one can look to research comparing the gut flora of children raised in different communities. Studies have demonstrated that infants raised in rural environments (where children have a lower incidence of allergic disease) have a predominance of a bacterial species known as *Bifido-bacterium* in their guts. Infants raised in urban areas, on the other hand, have predominantly *Bacteroides* species in their guts. This early colonization of the GI tract has major implications for overall health, including on the presentation of atopic disorders. As humans, we have coevolved along with our microbiomes (simply a population of microorganisms) to help us perform immunologic and digestive functions we can't complete on our own. If the balance of gut flora is disrupted at a young age (GI dysbiosis), children may experience *sensitization* rather than tolerance to a number of allergenic foods. Sensitization is an inflammatory allergic response that can occur after exposure to food proteins, and it can lead to allergic reactions upon subsequent exposure. In an infant with a healthy gut microbiome, those same food proteins would theoretically be well tolerated, enabling the child to ingest the food regularly without issue.

Multiple factors can lead to the disruption of gut flora in early life and trigger an allergic and inflammatory response:

- **Antibiotics.** If a mother has bacterial infections during pregnancy that require antibiotics, many of those broad-spectrum antibiotics can cross the placenta and reach the fetus. In addition, antibiotics can have a profound effect on Mom's GI and vaginal microbiome, resulting in prolonged dysbiosis. In fact, just a single course of oral antibiotics can disrupt the gut

microbiome for an entire year! If Mom received antibiotics during pregnancy, a baby delivered via vaginal
delivery will become colonized with a population of
gut and vaginal flora from Mom that has been altered
by those antibiotics.

· **C-section.** When a mother has a cesarean section
delivery, her child is not exposed to the population
of microorganisms that inhabit the birth canal (which
is largely composed of *Lactobacillus, Prevotella,* and
Sneathia species). Instead, the child will be exposed
to the population of bacteria that inhabits the skin
of the first person who touches him or her (such as
Staphylococcus, Corynebacterium, and *Propionibacte-
rium* species). Additionally, beneficial *Bifidobacterium*
species that are transmitted from Mom to baby during
vaginal delivery are not transmitted during C-section.

· **Lack of breast milk.** Breast milk can strengthen a
baby's microbiome. A 2017 study[1] from University of
California, Los Angeles found that approximately 30
percent of the beneficial bacteria in a baby's intestinal
tract come directly from mother's milk, and an additional 10 percent come from the skin on a mother's
breast. Unfortunately, not every mother can breastfeed successfully. There are a number of reasons this
may be the case: sometimes milk doesn't come in,

---

1   P. S. Pannaraj, F. Li, C. Cerini, J. M. Bender, S. Yang, A. Rollie, H. Adisetiyo, et al., "Association
    between Breast Milk Bacterial Communities and Establishment and Development of the Infant
    Gut Microbiome," *JAMA Pediatrics* 171, no. 7: 647–654, doi: 10.1001/jamapediatrics.2017.0378.

or illness and medication may prevent breastfeeding. Whatever the reason, a lack of breast milk can interfere with the development of an optimized gut microbiome in an infant.

From an evolutionary perspective, humans are meant to be born vaginally, to be breastfed in infancy, and to not be exposed to medication. Scientific progress has given society medical advances including antibiotics, delivery via C-section, and infant formula. Do these interventions help save lives? Absolutely. We must realize, however, that every intervention we perform in medicine has an impact beyond its intended effect. The solution for dysbiosis resulting from medical intervention is not to go back to the Dark Ages. Rather, we must look for ways to mitigate the negative effects on the gut flora caused by lifesaving interventions. The good news is that researchers are actively exploring how to design and employ methods to protect microbiome integrity, and the science is getting stronger all the time. The following areas of study can support mothers and children as they focus on balancing the gut biome in those critical first moments:

- **Minimize unnecessary antibiotics.** As more antibiotics have been developed, people have lost the patience to endure even minor viral infections without medical intervention. The truth is, when used incorrectly, antibiotics don't make our bodies heal any faster, but they do cause side effects. One of those side effects is GI dysbiosis. Therefore, it is important to use antibiotics only when needed and to employ a bit of patience prior to jumping to medication. Don't get me wrong—I'm not implying that pregnant mothers should opt for coconut oil or energy healing instead of taking antibiotics for severe infections. There are some scenarios in which antibiotics are both indicated and potentially lifesaving. Still, cautious use of antibiotics and selection of those medications with the narrowest possible spectrum of activity may help avoid inflammatory and allergic reactions down the road.

· **Vaginal seeding for C-section babies.** Vaginal seeding refers to the practice of swabbing the nose and mouth of a newborn infant with a gauze or swab that has been inoculated with the mother's vaginal fluid secretions. The idea behind vaginal seeding is to provide babies born via C-section exposure to beneficial flora from the birth canal, which they might miss out on if delivered via C-section before Mom's water breaks. Why is this important? The theory is that proper colonization of the infant's gut microbiome will help prevent the increase in allergic disorders that is associated with C-section delivery. In a small pilot study of eighteen newborns (seven born vaginally and eleven delivered via C-section), researchers attempted to study the effect of partial restoration of infant microbiota via vaginal seeding.

Of the eleven babies delivered via C-section, four babies had the seeding procedure performed after testing mothers and ruling out the presence of group B strep colonization or signs of vaginal inflammation and infection. Microbial cultures and testing revealed that the microbiomes of the four babies who underwent vaginal seeding resembled those of vaginally delivered infants, particularly in the first week of life. However, the study was very small, and no data was shared on the long-term health of these infants after seeding. Therefore, the current recommendation of the American College of Obstetrics and Gynecology is that vaginal seeding only be performed in the context of an approved research protocol. Future study will certainly be needed to help refine those populations of infants most likely to benefit from vaginal seeding and develop protocols to reduce the risk of transmitting infections such as group B strep and sexually transmitted diseases from mothers to babies. It will also be necessary to study the long-term effects of vaginal seeding on the health of children beyond the early stages of infancy.

- **Use probiotics.** For those babies exposed to antibiotics, born via C-section, or not able to breastfeed, giving carefully selected probiotics may help to introduce microbial species that they might otherwise be missing. These "good bacteria" can help to aid digestion, ferment unused energy stores, produce vitamins, inhibit the growth of harmful pathogens, stimulate the immune system, and regulate gut development. Not all probiotics are created equal, however. It is important to work with your physician to select probiotics specially designed for infants. These probiotics have a formulation that can withstand long-term storage and traveling through the harsh environment of the stomach and intestine. It is also essential to avoid giving probiotics to babies with immune deficiencies, as this may pose an infection risk.

- **Add prebiotics and probiotics to formula.** For babies who are not able to drink breastmilk, infant formula can offer not only nutrition but possibly also microbiome support. Some infant formulas now include probiotics to mimic the healthy bacteria children would be exposed to from their mother's milk, in addition to prebiotics, which are indigestible forms of dietary fiber. Why is including both the prebiotic and probiotic important? The probiotic is the actual microorganism, and the prebiotic is its food, helping it thrive.

- **Introduce fermented foods.** Our ancestors understood that fermented foods have health benefits, and many cultures have traditionally included such foods into their daily diet. Consider the prevalence of kimchi (high in *Lactobacillus* species, among others) in the Korean peninsula or the Indian tradition of consuming pickled fruits and vegetables (achar) with every meal.

In Eurasia, they drink kefir, a fermented yogurt drink containing probiotic strains, including *Lactobacillus*, *Bifidobacterium*, and *Streptococcus thermophilus*. Sourdough bread, sauerkraut, kombucha, and miso are other foods that introduce probiotics into the digestive tract. As the Western diet is high in processed foods that include preservatives and may be lacking in the nutritional value of homemade cuisine, adding some fermented foods to the menu is a reasonable way to introduce beneficial bacteria into the diet.

THE DUAL-ALLERGEN EXPOSURE HYPOTHESIS

Another potential factor in the progression of the allergic march is described by the dual-allergen exposure hypothesis. This theory suggests that tolerance to foods develops in young babies through high-dose oral exposure. It further argues that sensitization to the same foods can occur through even low-dose exposure through the skin. The critical point, then, is this: Which food exposure occurs first, oral or cutaneous? For a child with eczema, it's likely the latter, and it typically occurs before the baby has an opportunity to start eating solids and gain regular exposure to the potential allergen through their digestive tract. This scenario leaves the child at an increased risk of developing a hypersensitivity to that food.

Let's look at an everyday example to put this into perspective. Say an infant with eczema who has not yet started eating solids lives in a household where peanut butter and eggs are regularly eaten by his parents and siblings. Can the baby become sensitized to those allergens? Yes. The baby can be sensitized to those foods through his skin before being tolerized through the gut. How does this occur? Food allergens on the hands and lips of family members gain access to the baby's immune system by entering through eczematous skin during routine activities such as changing, bathing, cuddling, or kissing.

You see, the skin is the largest organ in the body and our first defense against foreign invaders, whether they be pathogens such as bacteria or allergens such as foods. Most children have a strong skin barrier with cells that adhere tightly to one another on a microscopic level, effectively creating a shield against the outside world. If a child has a genetic predisposition to developing eczema, however, the connections between skin cells are not tight and this causes the skin to be "leaky." Lipids and moisture escape through the gaps, causing those with eczema to have exceptionally dry skin that is prone to itchy rashes and infection—and allergens get in, precipitating food sensitization.

This dual exposure hypothesis of food allergy makes the case that it is essential to treat eczema aggressively and keep the skin barrier intact during the critical immuno-logic window in infancy if we hope to minimize the risk of food allergy. In addition, the hypothesis also suggests that the traditional advice to delay the introduction of potential food allergens to babies may be counterproductive.

LANDMARK STUDIES FURTHER THE CASE FOR DESENSITIZATION

The most disruptive (in a good way) research to build from the dual-exposure hypothesis can be found in the well-cited Learning Early About Peanut Allergy (LEAP) and Persistence of Oral Tolerance to Peanut (LEAP-ON) studies. LEAP and LEAP-ON's research were sponsored by the Immune Tolerance Network (ITN), a collaborative network for clinical research led by the National Institute of Allergy and Infectious Diseases under the National Institutes of Health (NIH). Both are landmark studies when it comes to investigating the development of food allergies in young children.

The LEAP study was prompted by observations that children in Israel, who are commonly fed peanut-containing snacks in infancy, had lower rates of peanut allergy compared to children in the United Kingdom and United States, where the guidance had been to delay the introduction of peanut until age three years. LEAP researchers studied 640 infants with a high risk of developing peanut allergy due to having severe eczema, egg allergy, or both. They randomized the infants into two groups: peanut avoidance and peanut consumption (six grams of peanut protein per week, divided into three or more servings), and the study participants were followed for five years. The LEAP research team found that in the group that was exposed to peanut regularly at a young age, only 3.2 percent developed peanut allergy during the five-year study period. What about the high-risk group that practiced strict avoidance? Just over 17 percent of these children developed peanut allergy, a significantly higher percentage than the infants— remember, with the same risk—who had early digestive exposure to peanuts.[2]

Essentially, the LEAP study turned the recommendation for dietary introduction in young children on its head, reversing the standard advice to delay introduction until arbitrary milestones. Dr. Gideon Lack, renowned UK allergist and lead investigator of the LEAP study, went so far as to say the decades of avoidance advice doctors had been offering was likely contributing to the rise in peanut allergies around the globe.

In 2016, the results from the follow-up study (LEAP-ON) were presented and published in the *New England Journal of Medicine*. The goal of this one-year extension study was

2   George Du Toit, Graham Roberts, Peter H. Sayre, Henry T. Bahnson, Suzana Radulovic, Alexandra F. Santos, Helen A. Brough, et al., "Randomized Trial of Peanut Consumption in Infants at Risk for Peanut Allergy," *New England Journal of Medicine* 372, no. 9 (2015): 803-813, doi: 10.1056/nejmoa1414850.

to determine if the benefits of early peanut introduction could be maintained without continued peanut ingestion. Dr. Lack and his team examined 556 of the children from the original LEAP study and had them all avoid peanut for a full year. Peanut allergy continued to be much more prevalent in the LEAP avoiders (18.6 percent) than in the LEAP consumers (4.8 percent). More importantly, there was no statistically significant increase in peanut allergy in the LEAP consumption group during the year of peanut avoidance. This suggests that when peanut is introduced early in life to high-risk infants, the immune system has the ability to create a memory response and maintain a state of tolerance. This is true even when the peanut is no longer eaten for an extended time.

Ultimately, LEAP-ON offered reassurance that eating peanut-containing foods occasionally as part of a normal diet would be a safe practice following successful tolerance induction. This proved true even if there were occasional gaps in peanut consumption.

A third study, Enquiring About Tolerance (EAT), examined the effect of early introduction of a variety of common food allergens into the diet of breastfed infants (not high risk) on the development of food allergy. More than 1,300 infants were randomized to either start consuming two grams each of common food allergens each week beginning at three months of age or to continue exclusive breastfeeding for the first six months of life. The subjects were followed for three years. The study showed that early introduction of two grams per week of peanut and egg white protein significantly reduced allergy. Additional analysis demonstrated that food allergy was less likely when more foods were consumed, with increased weekly amounts of foods consumed, and with an extended duration of consumption.

What are the key lessons from these studies? First, early food exposure in high-risk infants is associated with lower risk of allergy. Second, under the right conditions, the immune system is capable of creating a robust and long-lasting tolerance to foods. Third, higher individual doses and longer duration of consumption result in cumulative food protein exposures that are associated with lower rates of food allergy.

Although the three studies cited above examined children without a preexisting diagnosis of food allergy, the take-home points highlighted by this research inform the conceptual framework of treatment for children already diagnosed with food allergy. Desensitization, explored in depth in the next chapter, harnesses the power of the immune system to help these children live safer and fuller lives. It may not be a cure, but it is the next best thing—a *food allergy fix*.

CHAPTER TWO

WHAT IS DESENSITIZATION?

Sarah. Is. Frightened. She sits unusually close to her mother (perhaps hoping she might hide behind her?) as I introduce myself. At only nine years old, Sarah has been living with a milk allergy so severe that even a drop of it on her arm has led to hives and swelling. To Sarah, milk is poison, and although her parents told her Dr. B has a plan to help heal her allergy so she no longer has to be afraid, today, she is nothing *but* afraid. It's difficult enough for Sarah to understand the concept of desensitization, much less be willing to try it.

Milk is ubiquitous in our society, and for Sarah, it is a terrifying presence. In school every day, kids tear open yogurt packages, flinging her allergen all over the place.

They spill milk on the lunch table and eat cheese snacks that leave an orange trail of terror in their wake. All her life, Sarah had been told, "Don't eat this! Don't eat that! Don't touch this! Don't go near that, or we might have to call an ambulance to take you to the hospital!" The warnings came constantly, to the point she internalized milk as an enemy in her life. People stopped *just* short of telling Sarah that milk could kill her, but kids are smart. She understood the deeper meaning behind all the warnings. So naturally, Sarah harbored an overwhelming fear of the worst-case scenario. Now she sits in my office, her young mind focusing only on the knowledge that I'm eventually going to make her drink some milk. Sarah thinks this whole thing is crazy, and she can't believe her mother brought her here. As her mother tries to explain how desensitization will help, Sarah struggles to wrap her head around how she'll magically go from being all-avoidance, all the time, to deliberately drinking her poison.

As a parent and a physician, I know full well you can't *make* a nine-year-old do anything. A child at that age will exert her will. If she doesn't want to undergo treatment, if she is terrified, if she doesn't trust the adults charged to protect her, the treatment simply will not work. For multiple reasons, I will never force a food allergen into the body of a food-allergic child, whether it be in the course of an oral challenge or a desensitization protocol. I only perform these procedures with a child's assent.

Why? First of all, I want to respect the autonomy and self-determination of my young patients. I cannot establish rapport and a trusting relationship with a scared child if they are convinced I am trying to kill them. Second, consuming a food allergen in the context of overwhelming anxiety puts the patient at risk, physically. If your heart is racing with every visit to the doctor for an allergen dose, you are actually more likely to have an allergic reaction. By the same token, you can't have been recently crying or having a temper tantrum. You can't be overheated from exercise or have a racing heart from running into our office. To reduce the risk of reacting to an OIT dose, patients must be in a calm state with a steady heart rate and baseline body temperature. In order to comply with these safety requirements, and to ease their natural anxiety, it is imperative that children understand what we hope to accomplish with desensitization and how we plan to achieve these goals. Those requirements raise some key questions: How do you explain the nuts and bolts of food allergy desensitization to a scared and confused child like Sarah?[1] How do you provide peace of mind without glossing over the real risks associated with treatment?

---

1   With support, Sarah overcame her anxiety, and her treatment was a success. She now drinks four ounces of milk every day and can eat cheese, yogurt, and other dairy products without having a reaction.

A NUTSHELL VIEW OF DESENSITIZATION

My role in the administration of food desensitization is not only to design and oversee the treatment but also to put on my "teacher hat," explaining the process to young children in language they can assimilate and understand. In a nutshell (ha ha), I explain that we will increase the allergen dosage a tiny bit at a time over many months in order to avoid overloading the immune system. And as I always tell my patients, they'll start out with doses so small they would need a microscope to see them! This final point helps provide reassurance as the kids begin to visualize what food allergy therapy will really look like.

My favorite analogy when explaining desensitization is thinking of it as "taking your immune system to school" and retraining it. An allergy, I explain, is the immune system's overreaction to a foreign substance (usually, a protein) that, under normal circumstances, would simply be ignored or tolerated. To help explain this to children, I tell them, "OK, kid. We're taking your immune system to school because it learned something wrong, and we need to retrain it to learn the correct information." I use a basic math scenario to drive home the point. "What would happen if when you were really little, instead of learning that one plus one equals two, you learned one plus one equals three?" I ask them. "And what would happen if you practiced it wrong every day—one plus one equals three?"

I continue, "If someone asks you later what one plus one equals and you answer, 'Three,' they will remind you the correct answer is two. You might remember the answer in that moment, but if I ask you again the next day 'What is one plus one?' you'll probably say, 'Three,' because the wrong information is stuck in your memory."

I help children understand that our brains remember by practicing, just as our bodies do. "Now, if you commit to learning the math problem correctly and practice saying, 'One plus one is two' every day for months and months, the next time someone asks, 'Sarah, what is one plus one?' you'll say it is two. Practice makes perfect, and since you practiced it the *right* way over and over again, your brain replaces the wrong answer with the correct answer. Well, guess what? That is the same thing we are trying to do with your immune system. Your desensitization treatment is like a class for your immune system, and we are going to teach it that milk is safe."

When young patients are familiar with what the treatment entails, I present how it works in ways that keep them comfortable and calm. Here's an example of how I explained the process to Sarah.

"Right now, your immune system thinks that when it sees milk, it's supposed to go crazy. Basically, it says, 'Ohmy-goshOhmygoshOhmygosh!' It overreacts, making you itchy and swollen, making it hard to breathe, and giving you a tummy ache. But your system learned things wrong! Milk doesn't *have* to make you sick. What we need to do is slowly, slowly teach your body that milk is actually OK. The way we do that is to start by giving you tiny bits of milk, so small that you can't even see the milk with your eyes or taste it. I promise these doses are so small they won't make you sick. We'll watch you very closely to make sure you're fine. Then, you'll go home and take that same tiny dose every day. A couple of weeks later, you'll come back to see me, and I'll give you just a little bit more. We'll watch again to make sure you're fine. As long as everything is OK, you'll take that same dose at home for two weeks. Then, you'll come back and we'll do it again and again. This is how we'll take your immune system to school and teach it that milk is OK. By the end of this treatment, our plan is for you to be able to drink a whole glass of milk without any reaction. This will work because your immune system will have finally learned it the right way! It'll see milk and be like, 'Whatevs.'"

DESENSITIZATION AS AN OUTSIDER

I first learned about the concept of desensitization in medical school, but the discussion was merely an overview. You see, most doctors don't learn much about desensitization during basic medical training outside of being taught that it can be useful for patients with drug allergies. However, during fellowship training in allergy and immunology (the years of subspecialty training after completing four years of medical school and an additional three to four years of residency training), we really got into the nitty-gritty.

Allergists and immunologists must have a comprehensive understanding of the immunologic basis of hypersensitivity (allergy), which then sets the stage for figuring out how to reverse it. Allergy fellows receive detailed education on not only the practical application of desensitization but also the basic science that makes such a treatment possible—all the way down to the molecular level. This is all great, but the problem is that this knowledge has been applied only to the treatment of environmental and drug allergies, not food. Why? Until very recently, most allergists believed food immunotherapy to be too dangerous, especially because the standard method of performing desensitization was via injection, and there were legitimate risks associated with food allergen injections. A medical error in a peanut immunotherapy injection trial in 1992 resulted in the tragic death of an individual participating in the trial, which put an immediate halt to such research and training.[2]

Following this event, many allergists got spooked, and this unease prevented them from feeling comfortable even *discussing* food allergy desensitization, let alone practicing it. After all, we became physicians to save lives, not put them at risk! Injections in particular were considered risky because they had the potential of introducing an allergen directly into the bloodstream, which might precipitate a severe allergic reaction. Obviously, nobody wanted to be responsible for a patient dying from the wrong dose of a food allergen. The more prudent option, then, seemed to be to provide excellent education on avoidance and treatment of allergic reactions, and to equip our patients with lifesaving medication. Better safe than sorry, we said.

But here's the trouble: avoidance isn't foolproof, and kids were dying. In fact, in 2008, the year I graduated from my allergy fellowship, no fewer than thirteen individuals around the world died due to food allergy. Let that sink in. Thirteen lives lost. Because they ate food.[3]

---

2   Harold S. Nelson, Jennie Lahr, Rosemary Rule, Allen Bock, and Donald Leung, "Treatment of Anaphylactic Sensitivity to Peanuts by Immunotherapy with Injections of Aqueous Peanut Extract," *Journal of Allergy and Clinical Immunology* 99, no. 6 (1997): 744-751, https://www.sciencedirect.com/science/article/pii/S0091674997800061.

3   No Nuts Moms Group, "Remembering Those We Have Lost to Food Allergies," accessed February 7, 2018, https://nonutsmomsgroup.weebly.com/blog/remembering-those-we-have-lost-to-food-allergies.

It boggled my mind. How was finding practical protection from food allergies *not* the priority?

My interest in taking the leap to perform food allergy desensitization myself was piqued in 2009 after attending an educational seminar sponsored by my local allergy society, the Illinois Society of Allergy, Asthma, and Immunology (ISAAI). One of my colleagues from Texas, Richard Wasserman, MD, PhD, had come to present his group's experience with food allergy treatment. They had started performing food allergen desensitization a few years prior, and the results had the audience rapt with attention. Here was someone actually doing what we had only dreamed of and actually seeing success! I furiously scribbled notes until my pen ran out of ink and then made mental notes of all my patients who might benefit. At the close of the conference, Dr. Wasserman invited us to join his endeavor: "If any of you are interested in doing what we do, please reach out to us. We'd love to help you get started."

I was the only local allergist at the time who reached out to discuss the logistics of offering my patients this therapy. (We will not debate whether it was passion, keen foresight, or simply youthful zeal that prompted me to do so.) And true to his word, Dr. Wasserman's office was instrumental in getting me started with the practical aspects of food immunotherapy, such as supply lists, starting protocols, and so forth. I was gifted wings, but it was up to me to learn how to fly. So I modified and blended these OIT protocols with previously published research on peanut sublingual immunotherapy (SLIT; drops of allergenic extract administered under the tongue). I created my own hybrid peanut immunotherapy protocols, along with inclusion and exclusion criteria for treatment. I also developed my own hybrid (SLIT-OIT) protocols for other foods, including milk, egg, and tree nuts.

Why didn't the rest of my local colleagues also rush to offer food allergy desensitization? Many allergists were truly intrigued by the concept, but simultaneously, they felt uneasy. They saw the promise but worried that desensitization could not be effectively incorporated into standard allergy practice. They had concerns such as the following: Had it been studied enough? How would we ensure short-term safety? What were the long-term effects? What about Food and Drug Administration (FDA) approval? How were we supposed to bill for our time without a designated billing code? How would we build it into our workflow? How would we secure the staffing? Wouldn't we be inundated with phone calls in the middle of the night? Would we be sued? The uncertainties might seem overwhelming for a busy allergy practice that was already set in a routine. "Wow, this is really great!" they'd say. "But it's not ready for prime time."

I disagree. I believe food allergy desensitization is a

therapy whose time has come. I have confidence that fellowship-trained allergists are absolutely capable of offering this therapy and have it within their power to save lives. But there is one caveat: You have to be willing to structure your workflow and staffing around the therapy, not squeeze it into your workday as an added service. Food desensitization is time and labor intensive. It typically takes me close to one hour to perform a comprehensive history and physical on a new food allergy patient. That does not include time spent interpreting lab work and developing a personalized treatment plan of oral challenges, medications, supplements, and desensitization protocols for each patient.

If your office is already in the habit of conducting structured appointments with a quick turnaround, it can be challenging to retool your schedule to allow these longer, more labor-intensive appointments. Additionally, systems must be in place to be sure everything is done correctly, safely, and with adequate supervision. I work with a compounding pharmacy to precisely encapsulate doses, and my office double and triple checks doses prior to administration. All my SLIT/OIT patients have the personal mobile phone numbers for myself and the other health-care practitioners in the office, and we make ourselves available 24-7/365. Allergy has traditionally been somewhat of a "lifestyle specialty," but the demands of desensitization turn that on its head. Signing up to be on call literally all the time isn't a decision that can be made lightly. I actually stash portable battery packs in multiple locations, lest my cell phone ever runs low on charge!

The challenges I discuss above have led to a low rate of OIT adoption among allergists. In addition, with no established, vetted system in place to perform the practice and be compensated for it—or, importantly, have protection from liability—a new model can understandably be a concern for doctors. Early in my allergy career, working in an office that provided excellent allergy and asthma care but was indeed not yet ready for OIT, I remained optimistic. I continued to explore the idea, identifying patients in my practice who could benefit from desensitization. It paid off, as I would soon start my own practice and structure the workflow, staffing, and even the office layout around my goal of creating a food allergy treatment center.

GAINING TRACTION

When I started my own practice, some patients transitioned from my previous facility. One young man in particular had a wheat allergy that caused him considerable distress and lifestyle limitations, and he was both eager and brave enough to be my first food immunotherapy patient. I treated him over the course of six months, and lo and behold, it worked! He was eventually able to not only tolerate wheat but also incorporate it into his diet. I knew that food desensitization worked in theory and in practice. However, to see it help my own patient was so gratifying that I knew there was no turning back.

I wrote about my patient's experience on my blog, and word got out that an allergist in Chicagoland was performing food allergy desensitization. The administrator of a large Facebook community of families interested in food immunotherapy (see appendix) reached out to me and invited me into their network. This was back in 2012, and it was a dual blessing to be able to learn from the experiences of so many patients and families and to also be able to offer them my knowledge and insight. Groups like these are a testament to the power of social media in creating true support networks in health care, and the passion for food allergen desensitization among the members of these groups is palpable. There is no one more committed to expanding access to a lifesaving treatment than the parent of a child with a life-threatening illness.

Despite its advances, desensitization remains on the fringe of becoming a mainstream practice in the United States. The most recent versions of both the European and Japanese guidelines for the management of food allergy provide for food allergen immunotherapy to be offered in medical centers with extensive experience in its administration, as well as experience in the management of anaphylaxis.[4] However, the American guidelines continue to withhold support for food desensitization outside of research centers, citing the need for additional studies.

Interestingly, the largest trials to date have not reported on the safety and success of precision-crafted food SLIT and OIT, as it is performed in private practices around the country. Rather, the studies making a splash in the news have been focused on ways to standardize desensitization so it does not require customization to the patient. Standardization also enables the developer to patent and monetize what might otherwise be available at your local grocery store for a few dollars. Therefore, these studies have been funded by the companies developing the ViaSkin epicutaneous immunotherapy patch (DBV Technologies) and the standardized encapsulated peanut flour immunotherapy product named AR101 (Aimmune Therapeutics). The millions of dollars invested into funding research and studies make financial sense for these companies, as peak annual sales are estimated to be $2 billion and $1.3 billion for ViaSkin and AR101, respectively. As for the rest of us, we are almost exclusively dependent on nonprofit foundations and governments to provide funding for research on nonbranded desensitization pro-

4   G. B. Pajno, M. Fernandez-Rivas, S. Arasi, G. Roberts, C. A. Akdis, M. Alvaro-Lozano, K. Beyer,
    et al., "EAACI Guidelines on Allergen Immunotherapy: IgE-Mediated Food Allergy," *Allergy*
    73, no. 4 (2017): 799–815, doi: 10.1111/all.13319; M. Ebisawa, K. Ito, Committee for Japanese
    Pediatric Guideline for Food Allergy, The Japanese Society or Pediatric Allergy and Clinical
    Immunology, and The Japanese Society of Allergology, "Japanese Guidelines for Food Allergy
    2017," *Allergology International* 66, no. 2 (2017): 248–264, doi: 10.1016/j.alit.2017.02.001.

tocols—a process that, like successful desensitization, takes time.

Nevertheless, I think there is value in any research that can be performed on food allergen desensitization methods. There is, naturally, substantial excitement around the possibilities of effective new food allergy treatments. Medical circles online swirl with posts such as, "Have you heard about the food allergy patch?" and, "Have you heard about the peanut pill?"

While I don't aim to discredit those approaches, I will say that success rates with standardized dosing regimens (epicutaneous or oral) are unlikely to be as high in general practice as they are with the type of precision-tailored, personalized OIT performed in private practice. More than 95 percent of food desensitization therapy patients in my practice have been able to successfully continue their dosing regimens, and my colleagues in private practice have very similar success rates. This is significantly higher than what is commonly seen in treatment research studies, and there is a good reason for that.

Sometimes a glance at such treatment studies can elicit a response such as, "There was such a high dropout rate, and why did so many patients have side effects?" There is a reason for that, and it's not because the researchers are using bad protocols. Rather, in studies designed to evaluate the safety and efficacy of a particular treatment, researchers must use protocols that are fairly uniform and rigid. In other words, participants must undergo the same treatment if the researchers want to gain statistically significant results. While this strategy makes sense from a research perspective, it's not the best approach from a success rate perspective. You see, patients aren't standardized. Every food allergy patient is different and therefore benefits from personalized treatment. A one-size-fits-all approach will always have limitations. However, if each patient is being treated with a customized protocol and receives adjunctive therapy (medicines, vitamins, probiotics, herbs) individualized just for them, you won't have a standardized treatment to evaluate. It's a conundrum, to be sure.

In private practice, we are thankfully not bound by a single protocol. In fact, not one of my patients has ever received exactly the same protocol. Why? I'm constantly tweaking it at every appointment to customize their therapy. For example, I may tell a child something like this: "Normally, we'd be doubling your dose today, but I think for you, we'll do it a little differently. Let's do a 50 percent increase instead of a full updose, and we'll monitor you for two weeks instead of one. I'll also add an herbal supplement because you're having a bit more burping than I'd like to see." This approach gives each patient a custom-tailored treatment designed to optimize their overall health. Because I am not shackled by having to study the same protocol in all my patients, I can personalize each and every component of the treatment to give them the best chance of success.

This precise and personalized approach to food allergen desensitization is working. I have a small office where I am the only physician. Nevertheless, we have had well over a hundred graduates in just over six years in practice. I have colleagues across the country with larger practices who have over one thousand graduates, so our number is small in comparison, but each drop in the bucket matters! If I can treat hundreds of patients with food allergies in my office, and other allergists with an interest in food allergy treatment follow suit, just imagine how many lives we could improve together!

STAYING AWARE, STAYING SAFE

Given the promise of food allergen desensitization as a treatment and the relatively small number of allergists currently skilled in its administration, one might be tempted to research as much as possible and "take matters into your own hands." After all, it's just food, right? For example, some might suggest, "Oh, just give your baby [who has already experienced hives with peanut butter] a little peanut butter at home. Give him a tiny bit more every day, and he'll get used to it." In theory, yes, that is what we try to do, but to attempt it on your own would be playing with fire and would be a dangerous mistake.

To ensure safe and successful food allergen desensitization, you need a level of precision that's simply unattainable in a home setting. I will grant you that desensitization seems an intuitive enough concept. However, you cannot lose sight of the fact that under the right (wrong) circumstances, even a previously tolerated dose of allergen might trigger anaphylaxis. In certain cases, an amount of allergen so small it is not even visible to the eye could lead to a life-threatening reaction. So if your child already has an established food allergy, this is *absolutely not* something to try at home. It is a high-risk introduction of a known food allergen into the system of a patient who is already sensitized, and it requires the expertise of a physician trained in the intricacies of immunomodulation. **All food allergen desensitization should be performed only under the medical supervision of board-certified allergist.**

In the next chapter, I'll provide an overview of just how desensitization works. The purpose of this explanation is not to provide a how-to or DIY guide. Instead, I want to provide the background necessary for you to understand the fundamentals behind how desensitization treatments can help treat food allergy. Armed with that knowledge, my hope is that you'll be empowered to seek out qualified medical professionals who can answer your questions.

CHAPTER THREE

HOW DOES DESENSITIZATION WORK?

Believe it or not, many people first learned about desensitization from the insufferably evil mastermind Vizzini in the movie *The Princess Bride*. With two goblets of wine on the table in front of him, Vizzini rants and postulates over which one is poisoned, while his adversary knows both goblets are poisoned. In reality, Vizzini's nemesis, the Man in Black, had gradually consumed small amounts of the poison iocaine powder over time to immunize himself to its effects. So, to him, it doesn't matter which goblet Vizzini chooses. Vizzini, however, struggles with the decision.

"You must have suspected I would have known the powder's origin, so I can clearly not choose the wine in front of me!" Vizzini rationalizes. After much rambling and a switcheroo, they both drink from their respective goblets, and Vizzini promptly falls over dead. His rival—although he consumed the same amount of poison—lives and continues on his journey to rescue the kidnapped princess. Desensitization to the rescue, indeed! The scene in *The Princess Bride* is a hilarious pop culture example of immunomodulation.

DESENSITIZATION'S EARLIEST DAYS

Desensitization isn't a new science. In fact, desensitization as therapy is downright ancient. It dates back to Ayurveda, one of the earliest systems of studying health, which originated on the Indian subcontinent over five thousand years ago. In the ancient Sanskrit language, the word *satmya* refers to a diet or regimen that is beneficial for an individual when taken regularly. It literally translates to "wholesome adaptation through habitual change." *Asatmya* refers to a diet or regimen that is not, at baseline, wholesome or beneficial for a given individual. It is important to note that a particular food might be *satmya* for one individual but *asatmya* for another. (See the parallel to food allergy?)

In Ayurveda, the concept of *oaksatmya* refers to those regimens and diets that have become noninjurious to the body due to habitual use, essentially changing the interaction between food and body from *asatmya* to *satmya*. Please note: You are not changing the substance through this process; you're changing the way the body responds to the substance. Food allergen desensitization by another name!

DESENSITIZATION THROUGH THE AGES

Mithridates VI was a king of Persian origin in an area called Pontus, a Hellenistic kingdom in Asia Minor back in the first and second centuries BC. Mithridates is known for developing poison antidotes—his habit the product of a tumultuous childhood. As the story goes, when Mithridates was around thirteen years old, his mother had his father murdered. She then ruled as the regent of the kingdom. Mithridates was paranoid that he would also become the target of assassination. Fearing for his life, he went into hiding. While isolated, he consumed various types of poisons in small doses to develop immunity against them.

When he came of age, Mithridates returned to his kingdom, had his mother imprisoned, and took over as king. Throughout his trials, he became famous for having desensitized himself to a variety of poisons—including the highly recognizable snake venom—to remain impervious to assassination by poison.

Much later, in the late eighteenth and early nineteenth centuries, the field of homeopathy slowly took form. Samuel Hahnemann is known as the father of homeopathy. He was a chemist, doctor, and researcher disillusioned by standard medical practices of the day, which included bloodletting, cupping, and the liberal use of laxatives. Hahnemann lost some of his own children to the influenza epidemic, and this personal tragedy fueled his impetus to study other forms of medicine. He noticed that certain substances given in small amounts were able to treat the very symptoms that same substance would cause if given in large amounts. This led him to propose a theory of "like cured by like"—in Latin, *Similia similibus curantur*. He thought of it as a type of stimulation therapy; for example, to help reduce the symptoms of hay fever, he would give tiny amounts of a substance that would actually cause rhinitis if given in larger doses.

Although homeopathy has since been disproven as an effective medical treatment, Hahnemann's work illustrates a concept that still has value: we should eschew overly aggressive and invasive forms of treatment when small doses of well-tolerated therapy might suffice. Now, food allergen desensitization is most certainly *not* homeopathy, as we eventually increase to quite substantial doses of allergen. Still, it is interesting to note the parallels between homeopathy and the early phases of desensitization: small doses of a food allergen may help to relieve the symptoms caused by a large dose of the very same food. Things that make you go, "Hmm."

Interestingly enough, during the same period that Hahnemann was exploring homeopathy, Edward Jenner pioneered what is arguably the greatest medical advancement in modern history: immunization. For centuries, smallpox plagued society, mercilessly taking lives and scarring those whose lives were spared. As a teenager, Jenner was an apprentice to a country surgeon in England. It was common belief at the time that dairymaids were in some way protected from smallpox, but no one could explain why. Jenner noticed that milkmaids exposed to cows infected with what was called cowpox did *not* develop smallpox. He learned that exposure to the cowpox on the cows' udders was likely inoculating the milkmaids and protecting them. After completing his apprenticeship, Jenner went on to obtain formal medical training and continued to study the cowpox phenomenon. In 1796, Jenner met Sarah Nelms, a young dairymaid with active cowpox lesions on her hands. He pierced the lesions to obtain the liquid and inoculated James Phipps, an eight-year-old local boy, by scratching the liquid into James's skin. James developed a fever and discomfort, felt sick, and lost his appetite a week later but then recovered.

A couple of months later, Jenner inoculated James again—this time with the liquid from an active smallpox lesion.

Understandably, townspeople were terrified of what the outcome would be, but James did not get sick or develop any form of disease. Jenner concluded his process had protected James from getting smallpox, and he set out to publish his findings. Unfortunately, his letter to the Royal Society was rejected. Undeterred, Jenner compiled several more cases and privately published a booklet documenting what he had done. He called his process "vaccination," based on the Latin words for cow (*vacca*) and cowpox (*vaccinia*).

Jenner is known as the father of immunization and creator of the smallpox vaccine. Based on his pioneering studies, the use of vaccination expanded throughout England. By 1800, the concept had spread throughout much of Europe. Immunization is widely considered to be the most significant advance in the protection from fatal disease ever developed, short of modern antibiotics and hygiene practices. At the time, the molecular immunology behind the success of immunization was not understood. Now we understand that immunization is a method of augmenting the immune system's protective response to a foreign substance (by producing antibodies) so that an individual will not fall ill when exposed to that substance in the future. Sound familiar? Things that make you go, "Hmm," part two!

In 1911, over one hundred years after the initiation of

vaccination research, *The Lancet*, a prestigious British medical journal, published "Prophylactic Inoculation against Hay Fever." The article described the use of immunotherapy or desensitization to pollen to reduce symptoms of hay fever—what we now call allergic rhinitis. The study used serial injections of grass pollen extract to reduce an allergic patient's rhinitis symptoms over time. Over the next twenty years, the process was improved to have smaller incremental dose increases with more injections over a longer duration. They termed the procedure "hyposensitization."

Fast-forward to the 1980s: "immunotherapy," the new and preferred term for hyposensitization, became widespread. This was deemed to be a more accurate description of the treatment, as further research demonstrated allergen desensitization was truly an immunomodulatory therapy. In other words, we were directly modifying the immune system by downregulating the production of allergic Immunoglobulin E (IgE) antibodies, the antibodies responsible for mediating allergic reactions, and upregulating the production of blocking Immunoglobulin G (IgG) antibodies. We have since further refined environmental immunotherapy to optimize safety and efficacy. The desensitization process has also been extended to other allergies, including medications as routine as antibiotics and as exceptional as chemotherapy. Bottom line? We know today that desensitization is an effective, life-changing, and lifesaving procedure. The next step: food allergy.

THE NUTS AND BOLTS OF DESENSITIZATION

You may be thinking, "OK, so you've explained the big picture. But I need more detail. How does desensitization really work?" Fair question. Let's discuss.

Building on the foundation of injection-based environmental allergen immunotherapy, we have found it is possible to safely apply the concept to foods but *without* using injections. Instead, we offer the food allergen in the way it is intended to be taken, which is via ingestion. However, we aren't just giving random amounts of food and saying, "Here, eat some of this." Rather, we have created protocols to ensure patients are being dosed with precise amounts of food protein in a consistent manner.

You see, it is fine to give imprecise and varying amounts of different foods to a young child who has not developed food hypersensitivity. This is the traditional way that babies and young children were fed, long before we developed jarred green beans, baby food blender systems, and organic sweet potatoes in a pouch. Babies simply ate whatever the rest of the family ate, ingesting small amounts over an extended period. They gained exposure and developed tolerance to a wide variety of foods at an early age.

Once a child is sensitized to a food, however, we cannot be so free and breezy. It is not safe to recognize that a baby develops rashes, itching, and sneezing after eating a specific food and then simply keep giving more of it. Allergic reactions can be unpredictable. The first time, for example, a child may just get a rash, runny nose, or a bout of sneezing. The next time, that same child might experience a full-fledged anaphylactic reaction resulting in respiratory and cardiovascular symptoms. That is a very big risk to take. Because we cannot predict with accuracy what a reaction to a full dose might be, the only way to treat safely is to start with microscopic doses well below the predicted threshold for reactivity. We must measure doses of food protein down to the microgram level and, in some cases, fractions of micrograms. After establishing that a given dose is well tolerated under medical supervision, we then increase the dose in a very systematic manner over time.

Even when a food desensitization protocol is customized and the starting doses are low, there is a small but real risk of experiencing a reaction *at some point*. That's just one more reason any new dose of a food allergen needs to be administered under the supervision of a qualified medical professional with expertise in the identification and management of severe allergic reactions.

BABY STEPS

As mentioned above, oral desensitization protocols start at the microscopic level. We start by administering miniscule amounts of food allergen proteins that are invisible to the naked eye and much lower than the predicted reaction-eliciting dose. This subthreshold dose is tolerated by the vast majority of patients. (For those patients with exquisite hypersensitivity, we may choose to start at even lower doses, with SLIT, and build up for six months before starting OIT.)

After confirming that the patient is able to tolerate this subthreshold dose, we induce "rapid desensitization" by giving repeated doses of the food allergen every fifteen to twenty minutes, gradually increasing the dose over the course of about six hours. The patient continues to consume the final dose of the "rapid desensitization" at home at least once daily for the next one to two weeks and then returns to the office. We administer the next dose in the protocol under medical supervision and observation, and the patient then goes home to consume that dose for another one to two weeks. So on and so forth, dose after dose, until the patient is eventually able to ingest a full serving of food allergen without triggering an allergic reaction.

How is this possible? The immune system will have become accustomed to each of the previous doses, one dose at a time. Each dose in the six- to twelve-month protocol is a literal "step up," pushing the patient closer and closer to a full serving. The amount of food that constitutes a full serving will vary by allergen. For example, one serving of milk is eight ounces, and one serving of egg is a single egg. One serving of bread is two slices, and one serving of peanuts is eight peanut kernels. Ultimately, we aim for protection to the amount a patient would normally eat if they were not allergic.

KEEPING PATIENTS SAFE DURING OIT

Once of the major anxieties families have about the process of food allergen desensitization is that they will need to dose with the food allergen at home. Parents often ask me, "I can handle the dose when we are here with you, but how am I ever going to bring myself to feed my child peanuts at home?" I can understand the apprehension because we are, after all, asking patients to dose with a potentially life-threatening allergen in the home setting. To mitigate the risk, we have put multiple safeguards in place to optimize safety when administering doses at home. Of course, all patients have emergency medication (autoinjectable epinephrine, antihistamines, steroids) on hand at all times, as well as food allergy action plans that are reviewed regularly. If patients have asthma, we also assess asthma control at each and every visit and ensure that bronchodilator medication is at the ready, should it ever be needed.

Other safeguards we advise patients to observe:

- *Never dose on an empty stomach.* Ingestion of food allergens can lead to GI irritability. Having healthy food (complex carbohydrates, lean protein, produce) in the tummy can "buffer" the dose of allergen and improve dose tolerability.
- *Never dose with a fever (>100.3°F), or when over-heated.* Having an elevated core body temperature can increase the risk of experiencing a dose reaction. Rule of thumb: If your face feels hot and your cheeks are flushed, take some time to cool down first.
- *Never dose during active GI illness such as vomiting or diarrhea.* Viral GI illnesses interfere with metabolism and GI transit time, and can lead to delayed dose reactions.
- *Never dose if experiencing active asthma symptoms (wheezing, tight cough, shortness of breath).* If you are not breathing easily at baseline, you may not be able to tolerate the challenge posed by ingestion of a food allergen. If you are needing your rescue asthma medication, don't dose with your food allergen that day.
- *Do not exercise or participate in any activity that raises your heart rate above the normal range for two hours after an oral dose (one hour after sublingual).* Exercise increases intestinal permeability, giving food allergens increased access to the immune

tissue in the gut and potentially triggering a systemic allergic reaction.

- ***Do not dose in the first twenty-four hours of a course of antibiotics, or in the first twenty-four hours after receiving a vaccination.*** It is not uncommon to experience fever with certain antibiotics (especially those in the penicillin family) and with the immediate immune activation period following vaccination. Therefore, deferring food allergen dosing for twenty-four hours is prudent.

- ***Do not dose when you are upset, and refrain from emotionally taxing situations within the postdose rest period.*** Youthful temper tantrums and arguments among siblings have been known to trigger reactions, so we try to keep things as Zen as possible.

All these rules may seem onerous, but they are necessary to minimize the risk of allergic reactions and to control the dosing environment as much as possible. Hey, no one said the desensitization process would be quick or easy! Truth is, food allergen immunotherapy isn't a Band-Aid that we can slap on and ignore. The food allergy fix is a real lifestyle change that requires dedication and commitment in the face of inconvenience. However, ask any of our graduates, and they'll tell you, the sweet taste of food allergy freedom is worth it.

DESENSITIZATION, TOLERANCE, AND THE IMPORTANCE OF EXPOSURE

To help explain the importance of long-term allergen exposure to successful food allergen desensitization, let's grab some props: a rubber band and a telephone book.

If you stretch a rubber band over a phone book, leave it there for five minutes, and take it off, what will happen? The rubber band will snap right back to its original shape, powered by the elastic energy stored in the polymer molecules. But what if you put the rubber band back on, stick the phone book in a drawer for five years, and *then* pull off the rubber band? It won't snap back but will instead stay stretched out in the size and shape of the phone book, because the elastic energy has dissipated. In this example, you have essentially changed the structure of the rubber band by "wearing it out" over time. It is unlikely to ever go back to its original shape even if it doesn't go back on the phone book.

One can think of the immune system as the rubber band. In order to solidify the retraining of the immune system after initial desensitization, the body needs to keep seeing the antigen on a regular basis. If you successfully desensitize someone to a food allergen but don't require them to continue taking regular doses, the immune system will snap back, like a rubber band, to its default state: allergy. However, if you continue to expose the patient to the food on a regular basis over many years, the process retrains the immune system and creates a long-lasting memory response. Eventually, frequency of dosing can be reduced without "snapping back" and triggering an increase in sensitivity.

Some studies have shown that patients can take a few months off from dosing and still pass an oral challenge afterward. This ability to maintain nonreactivity to a food allergen in the absence of regular dosing is termed *sustained immunotolerance*. That said, the studies on sustained immunotolerance looked at relatively short-term cessation of dosing (months, not years). The general consensus among allergists experienced in food allergen desensitization is that the safest approach is to make sure our patients see their allergens regularly, which for most means daily. We are a conservative bunch.

However, if children regularly consume the allergen as part of their diets, taking "formal" daily doses becomes less important. Take milk, for example. Say we desensitize a child to milk, and that child starts drinking eight ounces every day. If the child were to incorporate dairy into their diet on a regular basis after desensitization—that is, eating foods such as ice cream, cheese, and pizza, along with also drinking milk on occasion—we may be able to forgo a regimented daily dose. Now, if that same child doesn't care for the taste of dairy products and chooses not to incorporate cheese, yogurt, or ice cream into the diet, I am unlikely to suggest a long-term dosing hiatus. We can permit a few missed doses here or there, but this scenario is not conducive to a full stop. It's all about exposure. You can't perform an exposure-based therapy, stop exposing the patient, and still expect to see the same benefits.

WHAT'S NEXT?

Now that you understand the science behind food allergies and the fundamentals of how desensitization works, you may have some questions: How do you know if your child is a good candidate for food immunotherapy? How can you describe the treatment to your child in a way that won't cause anxiety? What are the options for treatment protocols, and what medical issues do you need to address *besides* food allergies to improve the outcome? In the next chapter, you'll discover the answer to these questions and more as we cover what to expect during your initial consultation and beyond.

PART TWO

THE FOREGROUND: YOUR JOURNEY IN DESENSITIZATION

CHAPTER FOUR

YOUR FIRST APPOINTMENT

Amanda holds the office door open for her four-year-old son, Joey. She is visibly anxious as Joey drifts to a corner of the room to examine a stack of books. Amanda brought her son to my office, clinging to the hope that there is something we can do to help him. Joey is allergic to milk and eggs. Amanda wonders aloud, "Why? Why *my* kid? I mean, his grandma has asthma, but I don't get it, because his dad and I don't have allergies. I honestly just don't understand how this happened."

My standard procedure at the initial consultation is to ask families to dig deep down into their memories to help re-create a comprehensive history. I start by asking Amanda about her pregnancy. After all, we know the intersection of genetics and environment is pivotal in the development of allergies. Beginning our focus as early as possible helps identify potential trigger events that might have nudged a genetically susceptible individual (allergic genotype) into a child who actually goes on to develop food allergies (allergic phenotype).

In addition to pregnancy, I also inquire about events surrounding childbirth and infancy/early childhood. During this discussion, many parents in Amanda's situation often have "light bulb moments" as they learn for the first time about risk factors for allergy that have been buried in their children's histories. I don't ask these questions to judge or pry; instead, I am trying to identify specific events that stand out as triggers so I can appropriately tailor the patient's therapeutic plan to address these "pain points."

Amanda relates that her pregnancy was uncomplicated. However, Joey was breech and required C-section delivery when manual maneuvers couldn't turn him around. Recall back to our earlier discussion on the association of cesarean delivery with atopic disorders. *Hit number one.*

As an infant, Joey developed frequent ear infections and required multiple courses of back-to-back antibiotics. "He would get the worst diarrhea and diaper rashes afterward," Amanda recalls. Remember when we discussed that even a single course of antibiotics can result in disruption of gut bacteria for up to a year? Imagine, then, the impact of recurrent rounds of antibiotics on the still-evolving microbiome of a young child! *Hit number two.*

Amanda also shares that she had been advised not to introduce potentially allergenic foods into Joey's diet early on. This direction predated recent study results that have shown the opposite approach to be more protective. At the time, though, Amanda followed the standard advice when it came to Joey's diet: don't introduce milk until age one, eggs until age two, and nuts until age three. When we connect all the dots in Joey's history, we see clearly that Joey didn't have a chance to obtain adequate oral exposure to allergenic foods until after antibiotics had led to GI dysbiosis. *Hit number three.*

Amanda reacts to our conversation with a pained expression that is now familiar to me. "I always wondered if I should have waited a couple of days to see if Joey went head-down on his own, but I never knew his ear infections could have had anything to do with his food allergies! I feel horrible. Maybe I shouldn't have given him all those antibiotics or waited to start milk and egg," she laments. *Sigh.* Guilt is so incredibly intertwined with food allergy that I have often only half-jokingly suggested that a diagnosis should come bundled with a referral to a good therapist.

Obviously, I don't ask probing questions or highlight risk factors to make Amanda feel guilty or responsible, but we must have these open discussions if we are ever to connect the dots and create a full picture of Joey's health. I reassure Amanda that she didn't do anything wrong and that it is perfectly normal to feel responsible and start second-guessing choices that were made years in the past. But here's the deal: As parents (and as physicians), we all do the best we can with the information available at the time. Sometimes decisions made with the best intentions have undesirable downstream effects. We need to free ourselves of the burden of guilt so we can move on from "If only" to "OK, what now?"

WHAT MAKES A GOOD OR BAD OIT CANDIDATE?

So let's get to the "Now what?" part of this story. Amanda has the same burning question so many parents have for me when we meet for the first time: Can you heal my child? Is Joey a candidate for OIT? It's a legitimate question. After all, there is so much misinformation about food immunotherapy floating around that many parents receive inaccurate advice from well-meaning but ill-informed health-care providers. A few examples:

- "There is no treatment for food allergy; your only option is strict avoidance."
- "Food desensitization is not available outside of clinical trials."
- "The side effect profile of OIT is intolerable, and most patients have to quit."
- "Your child is not a candidate because he is too allergic."

It's like an alternate universe, where the only information about food desensitization that families have access to is from physicians who don't offer it, don't support it, and don't understand it.

The reality? Joey, like most patients with IgE-mediated food allergy, is an excellent candidate for treatment. As long as patients do not present with food allergies complicated by uncontrolled asthma, recalcitrant eczema, or active GI inflammation, they're probably good candidates for desensitization. And there is no such thing as "too allergic."

In fact, you might be surprised to learn how many patients are good candidates for OIT, especially those who start young. When you're younger, your immune system is still in the process of developing and hasn't become "stubborn" yet. It's more malleable and responsive to retraining. Think of it like a lump of clay: younger immune systems are like a brand-new lump of Play-Doh, soft and easy to mold. Older immune systems, on the other hand, are like the Play-Doh that has been sitting out in a container without a lid, cracked, less malleable, and much harder to work with. This is not to say it isn't possible, but the evidence is certainly in favor of early intervention—before the onset of puberty whenever possible.

Of course, there are some patients who are simply not good candidates for OIT. As mentioned above, active respiratory, skin, or GI inflammation may require deferral of OIT. Let's take asthma, for example. If a child has been in and out of the ER with asthma exacerbations, requiring oral steroid bursts and the frequent use of bronchodilator medication, this patient is *not* a candidate for food SLIT or OIT yet. Notice that I say *yet*, not *ever*. We can address the root cause of airway inflammation, treat it, and reassess. It could be that her environmental allergies are causing airway hyperreactivity and we need to implement aggressive environmental control strategies or aeroallergen immunotherapy. Or she may require controller medication to keep her asthma under control, such as an inhaled steroid, oral leukotriene receptor antagonist, injectable biologic, or any one of the other medications we have in our arsenal to control persistent asthma. Once asthma is successfully brought under control and remains well controlled, we can absolutely reconsider her candidacy for food OIT.

The same applies to uncontrolled eczema and active GI symptoms. It is not advisable to pursue food SLIT or OIT until these issues can be adequately controlled. Otherwise, you risk compromising both the safety and tolerability of therapy. Aggressive application of emollients, decolonization of bacteria, and the judicious use of topical therapies can be transformative and dramatically improve the condition of a patient's skin. The use of carefully selected probiotics, pushing oral hydration, and management of constipation and reflux is similarly key to help resolving any bothersome GI discomfort prior to the initiation of food allergen desensitization. Take home point? First things first. Managing any active medical issues must be the priority if food allergen desensitization is to be successful.

Even so, there are a few scenarios in which I advise against pursuing OIT. I do not recommend food OIT for patients who are receiving chemotherapy for cancer, immunomodulatory therapies for active inflammatory bowel disease (Crohn's disease or ulcerative colitis), or who have active eosinophilic GI disease. I have made this decision in my practice out of an abundance of caution because I do not want to exacerbate or risk interfering with treatment for a serious medical issue. However, for patients with inflammatory bowel disease and eosinophilic GI disease, SLIT may be an option if they're seeking protection from food allergen cross-contamination and small-dose accidental exposure.

WHAT TO EXPECT AT YOUR FIRST OFFICE VISIT

Wondering what you might expect to discuss at your first office visit and how you can prepare to help the visit go smoothly? Let's walk through it together. The consultation will generally involve taking a comprehensive history, performing a physical exam, and testing—in that order.

Being prepared for the questions your OIT allergist may ask you during your first visit is a great first step. Common questions I ask during food allergy consultations include the following:

- Was delivery vaginal or via C-section? Did Mom receive any antibiotics before or during delivery for fever or group B strep status?
- Any health concerns in the first few days of life? It is important to know if the baby was not well after delivery and needed to transfer to the neonatal ICU, for example.
- Was the patient breastfed? How long was breastfeeding continued? Was Mom on a limited diet while breastfeeding? Did the patient receive any infant formula (milk-based, soy-based, elemental)?

- Did the patient develop eczema early in life? How was it managed? Did anything in the diet seem to worsen the rash?
- Was the patient a fussy or colicky baby? Any blood or mucous in the diapers? Did the patient experience vomiting or reflux? Was any reflux treated with medication, and if so, was it helpful?
- Did the patient experience infections requiring antibiotics in the first year of life? How many courses of antibiotics before the initial diagnosis of food allergy?
- Is there a family history of eczema, allergies, or asthma?
- What is the patient's food allergy reaction history? I ask my patients to create a spreadsheet of reactions, organized by date. The spreadsheet should have the following information: food trigger, amount ingested, time from ingestion to reaction, symptoms, treatment, and time to symptom resolution.
- What types of testing have been performed to identify and confirm food allergy? Skin testing, bloodwork? Once again, a spreadsheet of testing results, organized by food and date, is incredibly helpful.
- What advice have you received so far? Strict avoidance of all foods to which the patient is sensitized? Cleared to consume items labeled for cross-contamination? Have any oral challenges been performed? In many cases, by the time patients come into my office, they may have already seen two, maybe even three, other

allergists. Families have often received varied advice and may be confused about the right course of action. In order to develop a strategy for the comprehensive management of food allergy, we need to understand the current plan and then build upon it.

TALKING WITH KIDS ABOUT THEIR FOOD ALLERGIES

After obtaining as much history as possible from parents, it's time to talk to my young patient. If the child is old enough or has recently experienced a reaction, she may have some details to offer about food reactions. If the reactions occurred when the child was very young, on the other hand, she may not have a recollection of any reaction. This is especially true if the family has been practicing total avoidance successfully. Either way, I've found children usually have clear opinions about how their food allergies affect their lives. It's important that I not make any assumptions about how a child is emotionally affected by the food allergy and give them the opportunity to share their own experience.

"How do you feel about having food allergies? Does it ever make you feel sad? Are there things you wish you could do that you can't do? Are there things you have to do that you wish you didn't have to do? If there's anything you could change about your life, what would it be?" By asking simple, straightforward questions like these, I get incredibly honest answers—sometimes answers that the parents have never heard before.

Getting to the bottom of how children feel about their food allergies helps us define our goals for therapy. My primary goal is always to improve the quality of life for my patients and their families. This looks different for every family. Some parents may say, "We just want to make our child safer. We want to reduce the risk of accidental exposure because we've had reaction after reaction. We're ending up in the ER too often, and it's so anxiety provoking." This is a perfectly reasonable goal, and we can certainly focus our treatment on gaining protection from accidental exposure.

Other families arrive with somewhat different limitations and hopes for treatment. Perhaps the child hasn't been experiencing recurrent reactions, but the limitations of the "food allergy lifestyle" still feel stifling. The child does not attend birthday parties or participate in school activities. She may feel isolated, perhaps to the point of sitting alone at an "allergy table" during lunch and being unable to socialize with friends. Bottom line: she feels *different* and excluded. In this scenario, the family's goal is to gain the ability to safely consume items labeled for cross-contamination and lift some of the lifestyle limitations. This, too, is an achievable aspiration. In all cases, I remember that my aim is not to satisfy my own personal goals as a physician; instead, the mission is to help children and their families attain the specific goals that will bring about the greatest improvement in their quality of life.

Occasionally, I will learn a child's negative feelings toward his food allergy are being exacerbated by food allergy bullying—a serious issue that is far more common than you may think. In fact, studies demonstrate that parents are only aware of food allergy bullying in approximately 50 percent of cases. Bullying is directly associated with decreased quality of life for children with food allergy, and the child's quality of life increases when responsible adults are made aware of the issue. Therefore, it is worthwhile to spend some time delving into this issue, as uncomfortable as it may be to discuss. A child may describe food allergy bullying by saying, "Kids tell me I'm the reason why we can't have any fun food at school. They say we're not allowed to bring cupcakes because of me." I have also heard more severe cases in which children take peanut butter sandwiches from their lunchboxes and rub them in the faces of classmates with peanut allergies or threaten to squirt milk on classmates with milk allergies. As you can imagine, such circumstances can terrify a child who has grown up being told that if he is accidentally exposed to his allergens, he might experience a severe reaction or even die. One of the goals of food desensitization is reduce the distress associated with exclusion and anxiety, but we can't address the problems if we haven't clearly identified them. Food allergy bullying is a well-known, ubiquitous concern, and it's one I watch for closely.

UP NEXT: A PHYSICAL EXAM

After obtaining a comprehensive history and identifying pain points and their associated goals for therapy, I proceed with a physical exam. This is a critical component of the evaluation because a detailed physical exam can identify signs of allergic inflammation or related medical conditions that might be flying under the radar. It is common for allergic inflammation in atopic patients to be so chronic in nature that the symptoms are essentially thought of as normal. As I explain to parents, children sometimes reach a point where they get so used to feeling bad that they don't know what it's like to feel good. And if kids don't know they're experiencing symptoms, the symptoms are likely going unreported.

For example, during exams, I'll frequently discover markedly swollen nasal tissue with postnasal drip and cobblestoning in the back of the throat. Cobblestoning is swollen lymphoid tissue in the pharynx that gets bumpy, giving it the appearance of a cobblestoned street. Both postnasal drip and cobblestoning can be signs of uncontrolled environmental allergy.

Although I may see these telltale signs of environmental allergy on exam, the patient may have never complained about feeling stuffy or having throat irritation. Similarly, parents may not have identified any problem because "this is how they've always been." The family has been so accustomed to their child's chronic state of congestion and drainage that it never raised any eyebrows. In these cases, I explain, "Your child probably has significant environmental allergies that have not previously been diagnosed. Let's identify aeroallergen triggers with testing and address them definitively. After all, if your kid is constantly stuffy, with postnasal drip and a sore throat, food allergen therapy is not going to go smoothly."

Other times, I find that the patient's lungs sound tight on exam. When this occurs, I'll order a pulmonary function test to look for airway obstruction. I also employ fractional exhaled nitric oxide testing, which can identify allergic inflammation in the airways. The tests may reveal active lower airway disease, even though the patient has not complained of wheezing or activity limitation from asthma. In this case, starting controller medication for persistent asthma can make a world of difference. Imagine a kid who couldn't keep up with classmates to run the mile and is now sprinting along with the best of them—and that's even *before* we get to food allergy therapy!

If I find that a patient's skin is incredibly dry with active patches of red, oozing eczema behind the knees and on the elbows, getting the skin hydrated and clear will be job one. Why? Well, purely from a practical standpoint, the patient will be far more comfortable when dryness, chafing, inflammation, and itching are addressed. Additionally, uncontrolled eczema can cause certain laboratory values, such as eosinophil count and IgE, to appear artificially elevated. If labs are drawn when eczema is flaring up, the resulting values may give the impression of food allergies being worse than they really are. Therefore, I always elect to defer bloodwork until skin is as clear as possible.

One might ask, "Doc, we came to you for food allergy treatment, not for a head-to-toe makeover! Can't we just get down to business and skip all this other stuff? Let's just get her protected from the thing that can kill her. We can deal with her runny nose and rashes later." Of course, it is tempting to jump directly to food allergen desensitization because it's the most pressing concern. However, experience has taught me that any issues we ignore now will only rear their ugly heads at the least opportune times. Like a marionette on a complex network of strings, everything in the immune system is connected. If only one string is pulled at a time, the movements of the puppet will be all herky-jerky. But in the hands of a skilled puppeteer, the orchestrated movement of all the strings in concert brings the marionette to life, dancing across the stage. Allergists and immunologists are the puppeteers of the immune system. We do not serve our patients well by having a laser focus on food allergy (pulling a single string) without keeping a holistic mindset. We'll be much more successful if we treat the whole person. After all, it's all connected.

LEARNING ABOUT THE PATIENT THROUGH TESTING

After history and physical exam, the third component of the initial patient evaluation involves testing. Over the years, I have developed a panel of skin and blood tests that is incredibly helpful as I create an individualized game plan for each patient. This includes food-specific allergy testing, of course, but also incorporates other values that paint a more vivid picture of how my patient's immune and endocrine systems are functioning.

VITAMIN D LEVELS

There is mounting evidence of the importance of vitamin D in the regulation of both the innate and adaptive components of the immune system.[1] Specifically, vitamin D enhances the secretion of anti-inflammatory cytokines (cytokines are molecules involved in cell signaling and are the basis of how the cells in our body "talk" to each

---

1   Iwona Stelmach, Joanna Jerzynska, and Daniela Podlecka, "Immunomodulatory Effect of Vitamin D in Children with Allergic Diseases," *A Critical Evaluation of Vitamin D—Basic Overview* (2017), doi: 10.5772/65072.

other) and suppresses the production of proinflammatory cytokines. There is even evidence that vitamin D may play a role in downregulating the production of allergic IgE antibodies. Consequently, vitamin D is a key marker in my "holy grail" of laboratory tests. It's especially important because children with restricted diets are at a higher risk of developing vitamin D deficiency. Although a normal vitamin D level is defined as 30 nanograms per milliliter or above, I aim for more robust vitamin D3 levels (40–70 ng/ml). It's in this range that I find patients experience fewer side effects during OIT.

COMPLETE BLOOD COUNT AND WHITE BLOOD CELL DIFFERENTIAL

A complete blood count (CBC) is one of the most common blood tests performed. It is essentially a snapshot of your blood—white blood cells that protect you from infection and mediate immunity, red blood cells that deliver oxygen to your tissues, and platelets that keep you from bleeding out when you get injured. I always confirm that my patients are not anemic before we begin therapy. Children who must follow restricted diets due to multiple food allergies are at risk for nutritional deficiencies, which can lead to iron-deficiency anemia. This can cause fatigue, poor appetite, weakness, irritability, and slow growth. It is important to correct any such deficiency prior to the initiation of food desensitization. Next, I examine the white blood cell differential, which takes the total white blood cell count and breaks it down into the different types of white blood cells you can have.

When interpreting the differential, I pay special attention to the absolute eosinophil count. Eosinophils are the white blood cells that are responsible for mediating allergic reactions. In addition to being elevated during allergic inflammation, eosinophils can also be raised by parasitic infection or certain blood disorders. If the eosinophil count is significantly elevated prior to beginning food desensitization therapy, I try to identify the reason for the elevation to target it directly. I may also suggest herbal supplements to try to calm the eosinophilia. I track the absolute eosinophil count yearly in patients who pursue food allergen desensitization. A significant rise in eosinophil count during therapy may indicate an active inflammatory process needing my attention, so it is important to establish a baseline level.

TOTAL SERUM IGE

Antibodies (or immunoglobulins) are large proteins produced by specialized white blood cells (plasma cells). The function of antibodies is primarily to bind and neutralize potential pathogens and to help protect the body from infection. We have a veritable alphabet soup of antibodies: IgA, IgD, IgG, IgM, and the allergist's favorite, IgE. IgE is the newest antibody to be characterized (1966), and it is the antibody that not only protects against parasitic infections but is also responsible for mediating allergic reactions. It does this by inducing the activation of mast cells and basophils (both white blood cells), causing them to erupt and release histamine and other chemical mediators of allergic reactions into the blood and tissues. Most nonallergic individuals have relatively low levels of IgE. However, in patients with active allergic inflammation, IgE can be significantly elevated at baseline. Less common causes of increased IgE include certain immunodeficiencies, infections, and malignancies. I explain to my patients that total serum IgE is a bit of an "umbrella" value—it doesn't tell me anything specific but rather gives me a general idea of the cumulative allergic load a patient is dealing with. So I can use the total IgE count as a rough marker for how "allergic" the patient is and how much work it will take to get his allergies under control. I also use the total serum IgE level as a reference marker with which to compare a food's specific IgE value. More on that next.

FOOD-SPECIFIC IGE AND THE IMPORTANCE OF THE SIGE/IGE RATIO

One of the most pertinent lab values for a patient with food allergy is the food-specific IgE (sIgE). In contrast to the total serum IgE, which is not unique to any single allergen, the sIgE gives us an idea of how much IgE specific to a particular food is present in a given amount of a patient's serum. The concentration of sIgE in the blood is typically described in terms of kilo-units per liter (kU/L). The normal state of affairs is to *not* have detectable IgE to foods. However, if you become sensitized to a food, we are able to detect sIgE to that food in your blood. At most commercial laboratories, the standard range of detection starts at 0.10 kU/L, and goes up to 100 kU/L. One might think that one's sIgE level alone would indicate how severe your allergy is. However, you'd be wrong. Some patients with quite low sIgE levels experience anaphylaxis upon ingesting their food allergens, while others with higher sIgE values may experience milder symptoms or no symptoms at all. What seems to be more important than the sIgE value itself is the ratio of the sIgE to the total IgE. As a general rule of thumb (but certainly not a hard-and-fast rule), the higher the ratio, the more likely the food allergen is to trigger a reaction in a patient.

Here's an example: Molly and Nick are both sensitized to peanut. So when we check their bloodwork, they each have detectable peanut sIgE. Let's say their peanut sIgEs are 10 kU/L. You might think both are equally allergic to peanuts, but that may not be the case. You see, Molly has a total IgE of 100 kU/L, but Nick has a total IgE of 3,000 kU/L (he has very active environmental allergies and some eczema that contribute to the high IgE). Molly's peanut sIgE/total IgE ratio is 1:10, but Nick's is only 1:300. Looking at the ratio of sIgE/IgE gives us a clearer picture of the fraction of total IgE attributable to a single allergen. In this scenario, Molly's high ratio might increase her risk of anaphylaxis with only a small amount of peanut ingestion, while Nick's low ratio may enable him to pass an in-office peanut challenge.

Total IgE and food-specific IgE values can change as a patient's environmental allergies and eczema are brought under control. For example, a patient may initially present with a total IgE of 2,000 kU/L and a peanut IgE of 20 kU/L. Once I get the patient's eczema, environmental allergies, and asthma under control, both of these values might drop significantly. This doesn't mean that I made the peanut allergy better without doing any sort of food treatment; instead, it simply means I reduced the overall level of allergic inflammation. The ratio of sIgE/IgE stays the same, but as the total IgE drops, the peanut IgE drops along with it. By the same token, both total and sIgE might bump up slightly during pollen season in an allergic patient. By tracking the ratio of sIgE/IgE instead of sIgE alone, we insulate ourselves from these seasonal fluctuations.

What's so cool about OIT is that it actually lowers not only the food allergen sIgE but also the ratio, providing in vitro evidence of reduced risk over time. As OIT progresses, we can monitor progress by tracking sIgE/IgE periodically. Checking labs too frequently doesn't change my management, so we don't overdo it. However, it is illustrative to check sIgE and total IgE at baseline, a few months after completion of food allergen desensitization, and then yearly to observe the continued improvement.

COMPONENT-RESOLVED DIAGNOSTICS

To further refine allergy test results, I utilize a relatively new testing modality: component-resolved diagnostics. While food-specific IgE tests quantify the concentration of IgE to a *whole* food (milk, peanut, wheat, etc.), component-resolved diagnostics dig deeper, identifying IgE specific to the individual allergenic *proteins* within a food. This granular information has implications for risk and tolerance and is an important consideration when creating a "game plan" for food allergy management. Sensitization to certain proteins in peanut, for example, is associated with a higher risk of anaphylaxis, while sensitization to another is associated with transient oral itching and likely long-term tolerance. Similar predictions about risk can also be estimated based on component testing for tree nuts, soy, and wheat.

Recall Molly and Nick, both patients with peanut sIgE values of 10 kU/L. Component-resolved diagnostics might tell me Molly has a significant sensitization to the components Ara h1, Ara h2, and Ara h3—three components associated with a higher risk of experiencing anaphylaxis.

Nick—whose peanut IgE is also 10 kU/L—may not have any sensitization to those three components but does have sensitization to the component known as Ara h8. This is important because the Ara h8 protein cross-reacts very strongly with a birch tree pollen protein and is associated with a condition known as oral allergy syndrome. Essentially, even though peanuts and birch pollen are not botanically related, the three-dimensional structure of their proteins is so similar that the immune system gets "fooled." The immune system "thinks" someone eating peanuts (or almonds, hazelnuts, apples, cherries, peaches, etc.) has just eaten a mouthful of birch pollen. Nick may develop self-limited itching and tingling in the mouth, which generally resolves after drinking water and eating something else. Once the peanut is digested, though, the three-dimensional shape of Ara h8 breaks down from heat and enzymatic digestion, and it no longer bears resemblance to the birch pollen protein. Therefore, our friend Nick will probably *not* go on to have any additional allergy symptoms beyond his slightly itchy mouth.

To Nick, I might say, "Wow, your labs are looking promising. Your risk of experiencing a systemic reaction to peanut ingestion is actually pretty low. Instead of moving forward with OIT, we should consider an in-office peanut challenge to confirm that you can truly tolerate a full serving of peanuts. If we are successful, desensitization won't be necessary." In contrast, I won't be suggesting a peanut challenge for Molly, especially if she has a reliable history of reacting to peanut in the past. Knowing that she is sensitized to the high-risk proteins—and that she has an elevated sIgE/IgE ratio—we can predict that her chances of passing a peanut challenge are quite low and unlikely to be worth the risk.

The information gleaned from component-resolved diagnostics for milk and egg is different than it is for peanuts and tree nuts, but it's also very helpful. Rather than providing information about risk, milk and egg component testing gives us insight into the possibility of tolerating these foods when extensively heated or baked in an oven. There are three major proteins in milk: alpha-lactalbumin, beta-lactoglobulin, and casein. Of these, alpha-lactalbumin and beta-lactoglobulin are what are known as heat-labile proteins. That means that when the milk is extensively heated, these proteins break down, and their three-dimensional structure changes. They become denatured—that is, the shape of the proteins changes so that they are no longer recognized as allergens by IgE antibody and consequently don't trigger allergic reactions. If a patient is only allergic to alpha-lactalbumin or beta-lactoglobulin, but not to the heat-stable casein, he may very well tolerate extensively heated milk, such as in a cake or a muffin. However, if the patient is significantly sensitized to casein, which maintains its three-dimensional structure even when extensively heated, he is still at risk of a reaction from milk in baked goods. A parallel pattern emerges for the major allergenic proteins in egg, ovalbumin (heat-labile) and ovomucoid (heat-stable).

Identifying the specific proteins to which a patient is sensitized helps us make data-driven decisions, rather than just guessing if a patient might tolerate baked milk or egg and hoping for the best. In fact, a patient who is not significantly sensitized to casein or ovomucoid might actually receive a recommendation to introduce baked goods into the diet as a means of gently desensitizing the patient to the food to which they are allergic. Why does this work? Regular ingestion of baked milk and egg may accelerate the development of tolerance to unbaked milk and egg, and make future OIT unnecessary.

TREATING THE PATIENT, NOT THE NUMBERS

Although blood tests are important tools to ensure my patients are receiving highly tailored allergy management, at the end of the day, I am treating the whole patient, not just the number. What I'm really interested in is witnessing the patient respond to therapy and watching tolerance increase over time. The nice thing about OIT is that the proof is in the pudding (no food pun intended). We can see what patients tolerate every day because they're actually *eating* it, so we don't have to rely on bloodwork—although the numbers are nice to have for serial comparisons. In other forms of food allergy treatment in which the patient is not regularly consuming the allergen, doctors are reliant on labs or periodic oral challenges to determine the therapy's efficacy. In food OIT, every day is a different oral challenge, and we are definitively demonstrating the patient's tolerance day after day.

TEN QUESTIONS TO ASK DURING YOUR FIRST VISIT:

If you're considering making an appointment to see if OIT is right for your child, here are ten questions you may want to ask when you first meet with the allergist:

1. What is oral immunotherapy or sublingual desensitization?
2. What is the goal of treatment?
3. What are the risks and benefits of treatment?
4. How do I know if food desensitization is the right choice for my child?
5. Are there any age or other restrictions? What other options for food allergy treatment are available?
6. How would we manage any allergic reactions that arise during treatment?
7. My child tests positive on blood or skin testing but has never experienced a reaction. Should we pursue an oral challenge before attempting desensitization?
8. What can I do to optimize my child's chance of success?
9. We already have a primary allergist close to my home. Will you work collaboratively with our doctor?
10. How many patients have you successfully graduated?

CHAPTER FIVE

THE FOLLOW-UP AND TREATMENT PLANNING

Lucas is a twelve-year-old with multiple allergic inflamma-tory conditions, including tree nut allergy—the impetus for his visit to our office. Lucas has significant environmental allergies and suffers from runny nose, nasal congestion, postnasal drip, throat clearing, cough, and itchy eyes. On top of that, he also has persistent asthma, which is unfortunately not well controlled at present. Lucas typ-ically needs to use his rescue inhaler three to four times a week, which is significantly more than what a patient with well-controlled asthma requires.

Looks like Lucas has a lot going on in addition to his food

allergies! It's time to dive into what comes next: developing a long-term plan for reducing allergic inflammation and preparing the patient for food allergen desensitization.

WANT TO WIN THE FOOD ALLERGY RACE? START WITH YOUR RACE CAR

As it stands currently, I cannot safely perform food allergen desensitization for Lucas without addressing his environmental allergies and getting his asthma under control. Alas, that is not what parents and patients like to hear, so setting expectations at this juncture is a key part of my job. Many families come in thinking, "We're not coming to you for management of our asthma or our runny nose. We could have done that at home. We're here to talk about the food allergies."

In these situations, I use one of my favorite analogies to educate families on the importance of tackling baseline allergic disease before embarking on food allergen desensitization. I turn to Lucas's family and say, "Fixing food allergies with OIT is like a race—a long, important race. Think of trying to win the Indy 500 with a vehicle that's on the verge of falling apart—low fluid levels, rusty chassis, and flat tires. You definitely won't win, and you might not even finish! You'd much rather race once your pit boss has ensured your car is in tip-top shape. Lucas's body is his race car. To prepare Lucas for successful tree nut desensitization, we need a detailed treatment plan designed to help control his rhinitis and asthma. We have to address everything ailing him at this moment and tune him up before we get started so that he's poised for a strong finish."

Skipping this crucial step is always a bad idea. Why? I can guarantee OIT will be a rocky road if other conditions are still teetering on the edge of control when we jump into food allergen desensitization. I can't justify taking an unnecessary risk of OIT marred by recurrent reactions when we have straightforward treatment strategies available to optimize health and improve the odds of successful food allergen desensitization.

It's critical to have a body as strong, fit, and uninflamed as possible before we start our OIT journey. We have already discussed some blood tests (CBC, vitamin D, IgE) that can provide us a starting point. In-office pulmonary function testing and allergy skin testing are also valuable items in our diagnostic toolkit and can easily be performed in the allergist's office.

For asthma, I perform baseline spirometry, which measures airflow, and fractional exhaled nitric oxide (FeNO) measurement, which provides trackable information about allergic airway inflammation. Based on the results, I may suggest the use of anti-inflammatory medication (oral or inhaled) to reduce airway inflammation and decrease asthma symptoms. Patients typically start responding to asthma controller therapy in a few weeks, but it may take months to gain adequate asthma control. We can see measurable improvements in both spirometry and FeNO as allergic inflammation is reduced and as respiratory function is restored. Once we do, we'll know it is safe to consider the initiation of food desensitization. Not every child with asthma will need daily medication, but all patients should be able to demonstrate adequate asthma control throughout the year.

Patients with active rhinoconjunctivitis symptoms should have environmental allergy skin testing performed to identify specific allergic triggers. Allergy skin testing uses small plastic "prickers" to introduce a drop of allergen extract into the very upper layers of the skin. Knowing exactly which aeroallergens are causing symptoms helps guide management in three ways: First, we can implement environmental control measures to reduce allergen exposure. Second, we can appropriately time medications so they're designed to start working *before* the onset of the allergy season. Third, we can turn to aeroallergen immunotherapy, a form of environmental allergen desensitization, which can be administered as sublingual drops/tablets or as subcutaneous injections. Aeroallergen immunotherapy is very effective at reducing symptoms of rhinoconjunctivitis and asthma and decreasing the need for daily medication. Therefore, it is often recommended as a method of reducing total allergic load prior to the initiation of food desensitization.

It's a key concept among OIT allergists: the effective treatment of comorbid allergic conditions improves the success of food allergen desensitization and should be prioritized.

DON'T OVERFILL YOUR BUCKET

I explain the concept of total allergic load to children and their families by using the example of a bucket. The analogy goes like this: You have one bucket. It can hold only so much before it starts overflowing, right? We will call this bucket your "allergy bucket." Your allergy bucket holds inflammation of all kinds, and our job is to make sure your bucket doesn't overflow. Let's pretend that your allergy bucket is 75 percent filled with out-of-control allergic conditions: a quarter of the bucket from your flaring eczema, another quarter of the bucket from your persistent asthma, and yet another quarter due to your active environmental allergies. What's left? You have only 25 percent of the bucket still empty. That's not much in terms of wiggle room, because we'd like to introduce a food allergen into the mix.

What happens if I put a food allergen in your bucket, filling it pretty close to the brim, and then you get a cold? What if the pollen counts are especially high, or your aunt Millie and her three cats come to visit? Your bucket will overflow, and you may start to exhibit signs and symptoms of allergic reactivity. This may manifest as any of the following: asthma symptoms, eczema, worsening rhinitis, GI distress, or even as an anaphylactic reaction to your food OIT dose.

So tell me, do we really want to go there? Wouldn't it be better if we just took a little time to get those other conditions under control first and punch a few holes in that bucket? If we start out with a bucket that is only one-quarter full with a combination of your well-controlled allergic conditions, now we have an empty three quarters of the bucket to work with. If you come down with a cold, get the flu, or if allergy season hits hard, your bucket will not overflow into anaphylaxis from your food OIT, even if some of the other conditions temporarily flare. The buffer created by successfully managing comorbid conditions gives us breathing room. I always tell my patients I want to have their buckets as empty as possible before we start pouring into them.

THREE CATEGORIES OF FOODS

By now, I've made it pretty clear that in order for food allergen desensitization therapy to be successful, we've got to treat the whole patient, not only the food allergies. Assuming we have already attained excellent control of rhinitis, asthma, and eczema, now what? The patient is feeling great, aside from all the foods she's avoiding. Well, it's now time to determine which food allergens are good targets for desensitization by looking at a combination of the patient's medical history and test results. Looking at the patient's reaction history, historical skin testing, and recent bloodwork, I sort the foods my patient is currently avoiding into three categories: sensitized and likely allergic, sensitized but likely tolerant, and nonsensitized.

CATEGORY ONE: SENSITIZED AND LIKELY ALLERGIC

When a patient has a history of reacting to a particular food allergen, and skin testing and bloodwork confirm that the patient produces IgE antibodies specific for that food, it's highly probable that repeat ingestion will also result in an allergic reaction. The risk of reactivity is further increased if the sIgE/IgE ratio is elevated or if the patient is sensitized to high-risk component proteins. This is the "avoid or treat" category. Without desensitization, continued long-term avoidance of these foods will be required. However, most foods that fall into this category are excellent targets for eventual desensitization therapy.

CATEGORY TWO: SENSITIZED BUT LIKELY TOLERANT

Sensitization to a food without any history of reaction raises my suspicion of a false-positive result. Indeed, false-positive allergy tests are the bane of many allergists' existences. Improper interpretation of these results leads to unnecessary dietary restriction, exclusion, and anxiety. However, if the sIgE/IgE ratio is low, and there is no recent reaction history, it makes perfect sense to undo this damage by reintroducing the food into the diet. After all, it is possible to be sensitized to a food but to also have developed tolerance, which prevents any allergic reaction from developing after ingestion. So why live a life of unnecessary avoidance? An oral challenge is the only way to definitively differentiate between being allergic and being sensitized but nonallergic. This must, however, be done under medical supervision to safeguard the patient's safety in the unlikely event of a reaction. I make a point of trying to identify as many foods as possible for which to pursue oral challenge. In fact, I have often felt that the quality-of-life improvements achieved by performing oral challenges may be even more transformative than with OIT.

Here's a common scenario: many patients who are allergic to peanuts have always been advised to also avoid tree nuts as a precaution due to the possible risk of cross-reactivity or cross-contamination. It's possible that skin testing results may have been equivocal or slightly positive. In reality, we can't be sure if these patients are truly allergic to tree nuts. After all, they've never reacted because preemptive avoidance has limited exposure. If we order labs on a patient in this situation, it may actually reveal IgE-mediated sensitization to tree nuts. However, the sIgE/IgE ratio may be relatively low, or the patient may only be sensitized to low-risk components. In this case, I would suggest that patient make a few appointments for tree nut oral challenges in my office. If I am able to confirm that the patient can ingest a full serving of the individual tree nuts without reacting, the "tree nut allergy" can be cleared and our attention focused on the real food allergies. It is possible, however, that patients will *not* pass an oral challenge. If the patient begins to react halfway through a challenge, for example, that food will be transferred to the food avoidance category, and we'll shift back to a treatment mindset.

CATEGORY THREE: NONSENSITIZED

If a patient is nonsensitized to a food, it simply means that the patient's immune system is not creating IgE antibody specific to that food. Blood and skin testing will both be negative. So why might a nonsensitized patient be avoiding a food? Perhaps the patient has always been avoiding the food because they were told it would be safer (e.g., shellfish). Perhaps they were always too nervous to try it in the first place (e.g., tree nuts in a peanut-allergic patient). In any case, the risk of reactivity in a nonsensitized patient is exceedingly small. Therefore, I typically clear the patient to introduce these foods at home.

OUTGROWING FOOD ALLERGIES

Just because a food gets categorized into the "avoid or treat" column, it doesn't mean it will stay there forever. There are certain food allergies children will likely outgrow, such as milk, egg, wheat, and soy. The natural history of these allergies is, in most cases, to spontaneously resolve without any intervention. As we monitor allergen-specific IgE values over time, we look for reductions year by year. Also, significant reductions in IgE to heat-stable proteins lead to expanded diets. Perhaps a patient previously needed to avoid all forms of milk but is now able to tolerate well-baked milk due to a substantial reduction in casein sIgE. In six to twelve months, she may well be able to eat partially baked milk in pancakes or waffles, followed by cheese and yogurt. A patient like this doesn't require food allergen desensitization. Why? Her immune system is already doing the work of building tolerance without any intervention from me at all. Why wouldn't I allow this spontaneous resolution of food allergy to take its natural course? If it ain't broke, don't fix it!

ONWARD TO THE NEXT ROUND

History, physical, testing, and lab interpretation—check. Now, we move on to the next phase: dietary expansion. The goal of this phase of therapy is to whittle the list of avoided foods down to the bare minimum necessary to keep the patient safe. Then we make a plan to target those remaining food allergens with desensitization. Remember, the only way to prove that a food will be well tolerated is to eat it. So grab a seat and loosen your belt. It's chow time!

To start, I want patients to start eating anything they can safely eat. That means foods in category three—those to which the patient is not sensitized—should be introduced at home. There are some cases of "analysis paralysis," where parents or patients are so nervous to introduce a nonsensitized food in the home setting that if we don't perform the challenge in the office, we know it's never going to happen. In these cases, I go ahead and schedule the in-office challenge. That's how important it is to expand the diet whenever possible and exit the cycle of fear propagated by unnecessary food avoidance.

Next, if there are any foods in category two—sensitized but likely tolerant—that warrant an oral challenge, I'll conduct those to determine if the food can be freely incorporated into the diet. During an oral challenge, the patient is in my office for two and a half to three hours. During the first 90 to 120 minutes of the challenge, the patient is given multiple, incrementally increasing doses of the food being challenged, around fifteen minutes apart. Between each dose, we confirm the patient is not experiencing any reaction and check vital signs to ensure everything is being well tolerated. The first dose may be as small as a few grains of sand, but the goal is for the patient to eventually consume a full serving of the food in question. After the patient has consumed the final dose of the challenge food, he is observed for an additional hour to rule out any delayed reactions. Provided this goes well, the patient is advised to continue consuming the food at least once a week, if not more frequently. If any reaction appears during the challenge, it is promptly treated. We can then discuss the options of reverting to avoidance or attempting modified OIT (mOIT) with a higher starting dose than standard OIT protocols but a slower updose schedule.

One other benefit of fully expanding the diet is the potential for regular consumption of certain foods to partially desensitize to cross-reactive foods. For example, say walnut is in the "avoid or treat" category, but pecan falls into the "sensitized but likely tolerant" category. Successful introduction of pecan into the diet on a regular basis can actually help reduce the hypersensitivity to walnut over time, given that they are highly cross-reactive with each other. This is a case where a successful oral challenge to one food can obviate the need for desensitization to two foods. That's what I call bang for your buck.

TREATING MULTIPLE FOODS AT ONCE

In the early days of food allergen desensitization, only one food was treated at a time. This was all fine and well for patients with only one food allergy, but it created a bit of a dilemma for patients with multiple food allergies. How nice would it be to be able to simultaneously treat *all* of a patient's food allergies? Groundbreaking research on multifood OIT has been conducted at Stanford University, in many cases utilizing adjunctive medications (such as injectable omalizumab) to improve safety when introducing a large number of food allergens at once. I also occasionally use omalizumab, a lab-created anti-IgE antibody, which binds up free-floating IgE and prevents it from triggering allergic reactions. I find it especially helpful when working with asthmatic teenagers with severe or multiple food allergies.

Essentially, adding omalizumab improves tolerability of therapy. However, it is only approved for limited medical indications (food allergy isn't one of them yet), and I don't believe successful food OIT requires it. There is a strong case to be made, however, that we should be open to utilizing all tools at our disposal to ensure the safety and expeditiousness of food allergen desensitization therapy. Omalizumab, and potentially some of the newer anti-inflammatory biologic injectables, may have a real role to play in achieving these goals, especially for patients needing treatment for multiple food allergens.

There are a number of factors involved in the determination of how to design multifood OIT, including how many foods the patient is allergic to and what those foods are. I find that milk OIT is most successful when performed on its own. I generally prefer to perform peanut immunotherapy before tree nuts, because successful peanut desensitization often opens the door for a number of tree nuts (almond, Brazil nut, hazelnut, and macadamia, in particular) to be challenged. However, it is straightforward to add peanut to tree nuts and seeds when performing multifood OIT. When I perform tree nut OIT, I cover for all the tree nuts my patient is allergic to in a single course of therapy.

It's important to remember there is no blanket rule regarding the treatment of multiple food allergies at once. These decisions—like most surrounding OIT—are made on a case-by-case basis. There are many variables to consider. For example, the age of the patient is important with respect to determining what volume of food she'll be able to handle eating daily. As a parent myself, I know it's difficult to convince little kids to consume large quantities of food, especially foods they don't like. It is important to remember that many times, children going through OIT have a natural aversion to the foods introduced during therapy. It's almost like the body's defense mechanism: in order to prevent a child from eating large quantities of the things that could kill them, many food-allergic children are "wired" to simply not like the taste, smell, or idea of their food allergens. In some cases, it can be challenging to convince a young child to regularly eat a single food allergen. Will this same young child willingly consume four, five, or six different allergenic foods daily? As Donnie Brasco would say, "Fuhgeddaboudit"—at least, for a few years. Older children are typically more willing to overcome their own aversion to food allergens when they have a clearly defined goal in mind.

Another factor that comes into play when determining which foods to treat during desensitization is the cross-reactivity profile of certain food allergens. Let me explain. The major allergenic proteins in certain foods are so similar to each other that if you successfully treat one, you end up treating the other as well. For example, I tend not to treat cashew and pistachio together because they are highly cross-reactive with each other. I treat just the cashew, and at the conclusion of our course of immunotherapy, we perform a pistachio challenge. Similarly, I don't treat both hazelnut and almond—I treat the hazelnut. I don't treat both walnut and pecan—I treat for walnut. Again, these are not hard-and-fast rules, but in the vast majority of cases, leveraging food allergen cross-reactivity makes treatment simpler for the patient and "kills two birds with one stone."

SETTING THE STAGE FOR SUCCESS

Everyone wants to know: What is the secret to ensuring a successful desensitization? If you have been reading intently so far, you already know what I am going to say next. There is no golden ticket, but mitigating for identified risk factors and effectively managing comorbid inflammatory conditions is the best way to optimize treatment success. Let's delve into this a bit further, and I will share some of the strategies I have been utilizing effectively in my own practice.

Of course, I want my patients to be as healthy as possible when they start OIT, and that means living a healthy lifestyle. To that end, I encourage them to optimize their nutrition—that is, eating as many whole foods as possible, including whole grains, and complex carbohydrates. I teach my patients to balance their carbs with lean protein and unsaturated fats and to avoid going for long periods without eating. Because OIT does trigger low-grade GI inflammation at first, patients undergoing food allergen desensitization often get "hangry" when they go without meals or snacks for too long. They need a bit of food in their bellies throughout the day, so I encourage stashing healthy snacks in the pantry, in backpacks, and in the car. Additionally, I advise they limit carbonated or sugary beverages and abstain from overindulging in fried or processed foods. You are what you eat, and no one wants to be a Twinkie.

Hippocrates famously declared, "All disease begins in the gut." Although not entirely accurate, there is a kernel of truth to this statement. As we discussed in earlier chapters, when I look into the early lives of many of my food allergy patients, I see critical events that may have precipitated GI dysbiosis. To compensate, I encourage all patients pursuing an OIT program to take a daily probiotic. I believe that the right probiotics can promote immunotolerance and also provide a bit of gut protection during the process of introducing new allergens into naive immune systems. Why does this matter? The initial introduction of allergens into the body can stimulate an allergic response, leading to GI discomfort, stomach pain, reflux, or diarrhea. Probiotics provide a buffer against these issues.

There are two strains of probiotics that seem to work especially well during OIT: *Lactobacillus rhamnosus* and *Bifidobacterium*. *Lactobacillus rhamnosus* is a hardy species, is safe to use in all ages, and inhibits the growth of undesirable microorganisms in the intestine. It is one of the most extensively studied probiotics and is thought to have systemic immune-enhancing activity. *Bifidobacterium infantis*, in particular, is associated with an increase in an immune-regulating cytokine known as interleukin 10 (IL-10). *Bifidobacterium infantis* has also been shown to reduce distressing GI symptoms in patients with diarrhea-predominant irritable bowel syndrome, a condition that has significant associations with allergic conditions.

Another supplement I use in my practice is *Nigella sativa*, commonly known as black cumin seed. In Middle Eastern and South Asian cultures, *Nigella sativa* has been used for centuries as an ingredient in cooking, as a general health tonic, and as a supplement. It is also used as a home remedy for asthma, cough, abdominal pain, high cholesterol, parasites, and even as an adjunctive therapy during cancer treatments. Pertinent to OIT, recent research suggests that the active compounds within black cumin seed may have anti-inflammatory benefits in terms of reducing eosinophilic inflammation. Recall that eosinophils are white blood cells involved in mediating allergic reactions and promoting allergic inflammation in the tissues. For example, polyps in the nose and sinus cavities are generally filled with eosinophils. In allergic asthma, there's an accumulation of eosinophils in the respiratory mucosa. In allergic skin rashes, you can see a large quantity of eosinophils in affected skin. Similarly, in allergic GI disease, you may see an accumulation of eosinophils in the esophagus and intestines. There is evidence that high levels of eosinophils in the peripheral blood may also be associated with eosinophilic infiltration in the tissues. So if I see a patient has higher-than-typical levels of eosinophils in their blood, I often suggest adding *Nigella sativa* extract as a supplement once daily. Even for those patients without eosinophilia, I often advise them to incorporate *Nigella sativa* seeds into their diet, along with ginger (antinausea, anti-infective) and turmeric (anti-inflammatory).

Of course, any dietary supplement, probiotic, or herb must be taken only under the guidance of a trained physician who understands how they work and can balance the benefits with the risks. Like every aspect of precision medicine, these treatments are prescribed on a case-by-case basis, and they aren't right for everyone. It is possible, for example, to overdose on vitamin D and develop symptoms of toxicity. Some patients shouldn't take probiotics because they have significant immune deficiency and may actually become infected by the supplement. Other patients may have baseline liver issues and should not take *Nigella sativa*. It's important to note that the examples I have provided above are the strategies I suggest for my personal patients after completing a thorough history and physical, reviewing existing medications and supplements, and ensuring that there are not risks from medication-supplement interactions. I do not recommend starting *any* medication or supplement without consulting your personal physician.

CHAPTER SIX

MAXIMIZING TREATMENT

Six-year-old Amir is a picky eater with chronic abdominal pain. He has multiple food allergies, so he has a limited diet at baseline. On top of that, Amir won't eat the foods he is cleared to consume because his stomach is constantly hurting. He has not been gaining weight and is falling off his growth curve. Amir's parents have brought their son into my office because they have no idea how to feed their child and are seeking solutions. From my initial interview, I learn doctors diagnosed Amir with constipation and recommended he take polyethylene glycol (MiraLAX). While this technique can help and is generally considered to be safe, Amir's parents reveal they are uncomfortable with the idea of giving their son the medication. They once read online that polyethylene glycol might be linked with neurologic symptoms in children, and they got spooked.

Although Amir's parents are obviously interested in desensitization, there are other problems at hand. At this point, I deliver the news that I can't even consider desensitizing him to food allergens until his chronic pain is under control. First, I tell them, we need to ease his constipation and get Amir feeling well. On top of that, he has to be willing to eat.

I mentioned earlier that Amir's parents were uncomfortable with giving polyethylene glycol for his constipation. I should be clear that I, personally, am not convinced that polyethylene glycol is dangerous when used judiciously. However, I have been practicing medicine for long enough to know that flexibility is warranted here. I have a responsibility not to my clinical algorithms but rather to the family sitting in front of me. If they are uncomfortable with a treatment and don't want to use it, I won't force them. If I have an alternative they are comfortable with that might work as well, it is better for me to encourage them to at least try the alternative. I cannot be focused only on efficacy without any weight given to patient and family preference. Optimizing compliance with a treatment protocol is only achieved if the program prioritizes both clinical results and respect for patient autonomy.

After speaking with Amir's parents, I turn to him and,

again, use my time-tested race car analogy. "We need to give your body a tune-up, just like a race car," I tell him. "We're going to get you raring to go with a properly running engine. When it comes to OIT, the gut is the engine, so we need to get yours cleaned out and working well."

THREE FRUITS FOR A HEALTHY GUT

One treatment I recommended to Amir's parents was an Ayurvedic digestive health tonic called triphala. *Triphala* means "three fruits" in Sanskrit and is a combination of the amalaki, bibhitaki, and haritaki fruits that are dried and ground into a powder. Triphala can be given as a powder mixed into warm water or taken as a tablet. The blend is not a laxative per se, but it improves the tone of the GI smooth muscle and gently promotes bowel motility. Essentially, triphala helps the gut push out accumulated solid waste instead of just drawing water into the intestines. One of the downsides of other constipation remedies is that if they only loosen the stool without addressing bowel motility, undesirable effects can include diarrhea and dependence. As an all-natural product with centuries of use in the books, triphala is often more acceptable to parents who may be concerned about long-term side effects of other constipation treatments. Amir's parents certainly fell into this category and agreed to give the triphala a try.

Within a month, I received a message on my patient portal

from Amir's mother. "I don't know what this is that you gave us, but it's a miracle treatment," she wrote. "For the first time in his life, my child is not constipated. He's finally eating, and he's no longer complaining of pain." Had Amir's parents stuck with the polyethylene glycol and administered it regularly, might he have had a similar result? Sure. But the fact is this: they weren't comfortable with it, which meant they were unlikely to continue it as prescribed. The solution? Options. Amir is now thriving. Because his GI issues don't distract him anymore, he has started to expand his diet and gain weight, and his quality of life has already improved tremendously without addressing a single food allergy. He is also set up for future success as we create a plan to tackle his food allergies with desensitization.

TUNE-UPS TAKE TIME

For Amir, as well as all my other patients, I try to meld together a holistic and systems-based approach to disease management. How is your body functioning as a combined unit, and how well are its individual components working? We have already established that tight control of existing medical conditions mitigates the risk of experiencing side effects from food desensitization and maximizes the chances of gaining effective immunotolerance.

How long does all this "tuning up" take? My answer: "It

depends. Do we want to do it right?" Funny, but nobody seems to like it when I give this qualified answer.

You see, many patients come in to my office pumped up and ready to jump immediately into treatment. In fact, we sometimes get requests to schedule desensitization therapy for a food allergen before we have even met the patient. (These requests are kindly, but uniformly, declined.) When I tell folks it might be a year or two before the patient will be medically ready to begin, I often get blank stares. Anyone who has spent time in my office knows that a blank stare means it's time for me to pull another analogy out of my bag.

I explain, "I know it is disappointing to have to wait for something you want so desperately. But good things, quality things, take time. You have to trust my judgment and know that what I am suggesting for you is only going to benefit you in the future. Think of it like designing and building your dream house, the one you have wanted your whole life. If you want a structure that can survive the elements and stand the test of time, you need to invest time into engineering (crafting a treatment plan), building a reinforced foundation (optimizing baseline health), and construction (carefully supervised desensitization). The order in which we perform these tasks can't be rearranged. You can't build a house and then go back in and add a foundation next year. If we don't take care of the foundation first and take the time to do it properly, the house you build is going to be very rickety. You are going to be investing your blood, sweat, and tears into this effort. Let's make sure you have something to show for it."

I empathize with the concern families have when I begin to discuss the multitude of boxes we need to check before getting started with food allergen treatment. After all, time is valuable, and so many patients with food allergy fear that they are running out if it, that it's only a matter of time until the next reaction. However, they typically come around within minutes as I start to explain the value of a methodical approach to preparing patients for desensitization. As the saying goes, "Things of quality have no fear of time."

INTEGRATIVE ALLERGY CARE

Rather than practicing strictly within any single medical tradition, I try to pull effective therapies from multiple disciplines. These disciplines include allopathic medicine, functional medicine, Ayurveda, herbalism, and mind-body medicine. An integrative approach takes the best from each discipline and gives my patients the best chances of success.

Functional medicine emphasizes the importance of a well-balanced microbiome. As I discussed earlier, we initially get our population of gut bacteria from our mothers when we pass through the birth canal. As a species, we have coevolved with these bacteria over millions of years, and some of our digestive and immunologic functions are actually facilitated by GI microorganisms. When we do not have the right population of bacteria in our gut or develop GI dysbiosis, we cannot adequately perform these functions, such as fully breaking down our food or developing tolerance for food proteins.

We have already discussed events in early life that can contribute to an imbalance of organisms in the gut. However, not all GI dysbiosis originates at or shortly after birth. The food we eat can also contribute to disrupted gut flora. If you examine the food we eat now compared to the food that humans ate hundreds of years ago, our habits are extraordinarily different. So much of our food today comes out of a box instead of the ground. The nutritional value of these processed foods is not the same as eating whole foods. Therefore, we may not be introducing the right nutrients into our guts to help feed and maintain a thriving population of beneficial bacteria. Of course, the best defense is to optimize nutrition. However, it can also be useful to include prebiotics along with a probiotic supplement.

It might be tempting to assume that the easy solution for all atopic patients with GI irregularity or discomfort would be to throw some probiotics and prebiotics at them. However, we can't rush to that conclusion. GI discomfort may be a result of dysbiosis, but it can also be caused by other issues, including enzyme deficiency, irregular elimination habits, poor hydration, or regular consumption of a previously unrecognized allergen. How do we differentiate?

Sometimes the answer to this vital question is not immediately clear. Once I have ruled out other conditions, I ask my patients with active GI symptoms or rashes to keep a food diary for a few months. A paper notebook or digital spreadsheet will both get the job done. As we track dietary intake and compare it to symptoms, we may be able to make temporal connections between certain foods and GI complaints. A short trial of limiting/eliminating the foods identified in the diary can result in symptom resolution. Interestingly, the foods identified in this process often test negative on skin prick testing or bloodwork. This is because the allergy to the food may not be the classic, IgE-mediated type of hypersensitivity. Rather, a number of the foods that trigger chronic GI pain and/or cutaneous inflammation are delayed food allergens, mediated by the T cells of the immune system rather than antibodies. In my practice, I have found that food atopy patch testing can help to confirm some of these cell-mediated food allergies. Food atopy patch testing involves exposing the skin to small amounts of foods (in paste form) for forty-eight hours continuously and checking the skin for reactivity another twenty-four hours later. Although food allergens causing delayed hypersensitivity reactions are not candidates for desensitization, limiting foods that test positive can significantly improve symptoms and quality of life.

Enzyme deficiency can present with abdominal pain, bloating, flatulence, and diarrhea after eating but does not trigger life-threatening reactions. In these cases, pre-/probiotics and targeted use of digestive enzymes can help support gut function and reduce distress. My belief is that most patients with a healthy diet and balanced gut flora will not need long-term daily supplementation of digestive enzymes. Digestive enzymes are a temporary support until patients can rebuild a healthy population of gut microorganisms and find the right diet that works for their bodies.

THE AYURVEDIC ADVANTAGE

The term *Ayurveda* means "science of life"; *ayur* means "life" and *veda* means "science" in Sanskrit. Originating in the Indian subcontinent, Ayurvedic medicine is one of the world's oldest holistic healing systems based on the belief that health and wellness depend on a balance of mind, body, and spirit. The science of Ayurveda focuses on bringing the body back into balance so it can heal itself.

Similar to traditional Chinese medicine, an essential pillar of Ayurvedic medicine is diet, or *ahara*. The belief is that if you are not properly breaking down your diet, absorbing the nutrients from your diet, or eliminating waste products from your food, you cannot effectively maintain a state of good health. In the tradition of Ayurveda, there is a concept known as *agni*, which is loosely translated as "digestive fire." The quantity of *agni* changes throughout the day for all people, but the strength of your own digestive fire is unique. We can increase the potency of that fire or dampen it if need be. The goal is to optimize *agni* so your food can be properly digested. For example, if your digestive fire is weak, you will have poor digestion and possibly malabsorption. On the other hand, if *agni* is too strong, one might experience uncomfortable symptoms of reflux.

In Ayurveda, there are four different states of *agni* that point to different metabolic tendencies. The first, *vishama agni* (irregular metabolism), describes someone with an irregular appetite and signs of variable hunger, bloating, indigestion, cramping, constipation (or alternating constipation and diarrhea), dry stool, and frequent gas. The second, *tikshna agni* (hypermetabolism), describes someone with intense hunger but poor digestion. These patients are inclined to have a persistently dry mouth and throat, loose stools, hyperacidity, and a burning sensation in their gut. The third, *manda agni* (hypometabolism), describes someone who is anchored by weak hunger and slow digestion. After meals, for example, these patients often feel heavy and have sluggish bowels. Their stool can be bulky, and they crave sweets and other stimulating foods such as caffeine. The fourth, *sama agni* (balanced metabolism), describes someone with the type of digestive status I want to see. This is a patient with a balanced appetite and relatively good digestion. They feel like they fully digest food within about four hours of eating. They do not have any odd cravings for food or aversion to any particular type of food. Overall, they feel quite healthy. Alas, it is not common to find patients with *sama agni*. Most patients will identify with one of the other types of *agni*. Luckily, Ayurveda offers strategies for addressing imbalanced *agni*.

I sometimes turn to the four states of *agni* to help shape a personalized treatment plan for patients, which can include establishing a routine for daily activity, meal planning, and herbal supplements. However, I don't consider myself to be an Ayurvedic practitioner, so I do not adhere strictly to the traditional dietary prescriptions, which can be difficult to follow long term. What I choose to do, however, is to take some of the Ayurvedic remedies and use them where I think they can be helpful for patients. I think it is possible to do this effectively even without subscribing to the entire philosophy of Ayurveda. I firmly believe we can pull the best from a variety of medical traditions and combine them into an integrated approach without taking a religious approach to any single medical philosophy.

EXAMINING ELIMINATION HABITS

Proper waste elimination habits are crucial to overall health, and hydration plays a substantial role in maintaining healthy voiding. One of the things I have noticed over the years is that children are drinking less and less water. Many times, when I ask exactly how much my patients are drinking, I learn there are simply not many chances in the day for them to drink water due to modern school scheduling. Some schools do not even allow children to have water at their desk. For example, the only times a child might drink water are in the morning before they go to school, at lunchtime, after recess, and then after they come home. That is not enough water in relation to general health needs, and such a lack of water can lead to dehydration and constipation.

I am straightforward with children when discussing water intake in relation to elimination. I say, "I'm going to start asking you some questions now that might make you a little bit uncomfortable, but I need to know about your poop and your pee." Of course, they laugh and get a little embarrassed. "It's important," I say. "If I don't know what's going on inside you, I can't really help you. Let's talk about it a little bit. How many times a day are you going to the bathroom to pee?"

After they tell me, I ask, "Have you ever looked at your pee?" Then they look at me like I'm crazy. "It's important because I need to know if your pee looks like apple juice or lemonade," I explain. "Apple juice pee is no good. That means you're not drinking enough water. When you're well hydrated, your pee should be the color of lemonade or even lighter." When I explain it in this easy-to-visualize way, it gives the child a simple metric to follow to gauge hydration.

I often use the visual approach with children, even when it comes to discussing their bowel movements. Specifically, I use the Bristol Stool Scale, a diagnostic tool classifying human feces into categories, ranging from constipation to diarrhea. Developed at the British Royal Infirmary in 1997, the scale is widely used among gastroenterologists.

I use a somewhat hilarious variation of the Bristol scale showing anthropomorphized poop with superimposed sad and smiley faces.[1] I have children point to the image that most closely resembles their bowel movements. Occasionally, they are incredulous. "I don't know. I don't look at my poop!" If this happens, I ask them to examine their stool and tell me the next time they visit my office. If the results are types three or four (smooth, well-formed stool), I'm happy. If the results are type one or two (dry, hard

---

1   "What Your Poop Says about Your Health (For Serious)," *Mama Natural*, March 22, 2018, accessed May 23, 2018, https://www.mamanatural.com/great-poop-looks-like/.

stool), I know the patient needs to be drinking more water or maybe needs triphala or magnesium supplementation. If the results are type five, six, or seven (loose, unformed stool), I need to figure out why what they consume is passing through their system so quickly. For example, I might need to ensure they are on a robust probiotic to help improve their digestion or look at the use of a digestive enzyme for a short time until they can get their digestion issues under control.

THE MIND-BODY CONNECTION

Attention to psychological health is an integral component of an effective holistic treatment program. The reality is that many patients have been emotionally affected by their food allergy diagnosis. For example, some have experienced recurrent episodes of systemic anaphylaxis, requiring acute administration of injectable epinephrine, ambulance rides, and ER visits. This can be incredibly traumatic for a young child and also for the child's parents. Significant levels of food-related anxiety and even posttraumatic stress disorder (PTSD) can result. Even for those patients who have never experienced an anaphylactic event, the constant warnings and deep-seated fear about the possibility of a reaction occurring at any time can create a baseline level of apprehension that interferes with the enjoyment of day-to-day life.

Of course, food allergen desensitization is designed to

help allay these fears. However, we can't gloss over anxiety or isolation and wait until desensitization is complete before paying attention to the mental and emotional health of our patients. Understanding my young patients' concerns is a critical part of my job. After all, fear and anxiety are often the impetus for pursuing food allergen desensitization in the first place. Failing to thoughtfully address emotional health in advance will make the whole process of desensitization a series of microtraumas for an anxious patient, potentially compounding any preexisting anxiety. It is possible that these same patients will not tolerate desensitization because anytime they feel *anything* slightly out of the ordinary, they will assume it's a reaction to their treatment. Many times, the physical signs and symptoms of anxiety (uneasiness, heart racing, flushing, dizziness) overlap with those of an allergic reaction. This will create confusion among caregivers, who become stressed by the challenge of constantly distinguishing between anxiety and allergy.

To help my patients cope with anxiety, I encourage visualization activities, mindfulness exercises, meditation, and yoga. I also place emphasis on the importance of a consistent bedtime and recommend they eliminate electronic distractions at night in order to get a good night's sleep.

However, there are times when these measures are not enough. A patient may require the specialized expertise of a therapist, psychologist, or even a psychiatrist to address deeply rooted anxieties and trauma from a history of recurrent reactions. Sometimes patients are already on medications prescribed to them by qualified, board-certified medical professionals to help address depression, anxiety, and similar conditions. I don't prescribe these medicines myself, but I do work collaboratively with my colleagues with expertise in these areas to make sure the emotional well-being of my patients is prioritized.

It is a common fear of children visiting me for the first time that I will force them to start ingesting their food allergen before they are ready to do so. I take as long as necessary to reassure my patients that this will never happen. I promise all my patients: "I will never, ever force you to consume your allergen. This is ultimately your decision. Your parents want this for you because they want you to be safe, and I want this for you because I want you to be safe. What we *don't* want is to make you scared every day. This treatment only works if you want it for yourself. If you don't want it right now because you're scared or need more information, or just need more time, we need to work on that first."

Years of practice have instilled in me a healthy respect for the power of the mind-body connection, even if we can't fully explain it. Luckily, each year brings additional evidence supporting the interplay of the immune and nervous systems. We know that mast cells, the white blood cells responsible for mediating the symptoms of many allergic reactions, tend to aggregate at nerve endings. This means there is an extremely close connection between the neurologic system and the immune system. In fact, a 2017 study demonstrated that mind-body training was associated with an increase in the anti-inflammatory IL-10 cytokine.[2] Wisdom would have us recognize the potential of the nervous system to affect the proper functioning of the immune system and vice versa.

A RECIPE FOR THE ROAD

I try to employ safe and effective herbal remedies as an alternative to medications when reasonable. For patients struggling with burping and bloating after meals, I find that a homemade digestive tea can offer significant relief. Below is my recipe for digestion tea, a combination of bishop's weed, fennel seeds, and mint. If you can't drink a whole cup, just a few teaspoons after each meal can help eliminate excess gas. The tea is best when freshly brewed but can be stored in the fridge for a few days. As always, consult with your personal physician to ensure that it is safe for you to drink herbal teas before trying this recipe at home.

2 J. H. Jang, H. Y. Park, U. S. Lee, K. J. Lee, and D. H. Kang, "Effects of Mind-Body Training on Cytokines and Their Interactions with Catecholamines." *Psychiatry investigation*, July 2017, accessed February 26, 2018, https://www.ncbi.nlm.nih.gov/pubmed/28845176.

DR. B'S DIGESTIVE TEA

Ingredients:

4 cups cold water

1 tsp organic carom seeds – Carom seeds are also known as bishop's weed and may be available in your local South Asian market labeled as "Ajwain." The high concentration of thymol in carom seed makes it smell similar to thyme. Try lightly toasting the seeds on low heat before boiling to "soften" the flavor.

2 tsp organic fennel seeds – Fennel seeds have long been used as a carminative to reduce flatulence and indigestion, and have a pleasant, licorice-like flavor. Pregnant women should not consume large quantities of fennel, so if you are pregnant or trying to conceive, limit your consumption of this tea to the occasional cup.

10 fresh mint leaves – It is very easy to grow your own organic mint in containers. Take care not to plant mint directly in the ground, as it will take over your garden in no time. Dried mint leaves may be used as an alternative.

Freshly squeezed lemon juice to taste – Tip: Warm your lemons by rolling them on the counter or soaking in hot water for a few minutes before squeezing to help them release more juice. The juice will keep in your refrigerator for a few days. If you don't have fresh lemons, you can use a bottled lemon juice that does not contain any added preservatives.

Raw sugar, jaggery, or agave nectar to taste – Ayurvedic tradition cautions against the heating of honey beyond 104°F, so it has not been used in this recipe for a boiled hot tea. If you enjoy honey, a great way to incorporate it is mixing a spoonful of honey and fresh lemon juice to taste in a glass of warm (not hot) water and drinking each morning before breakfast.

Directions:

Heat the water on the stovetop in a non-Teflon-coated pot.

Add the carom seed, fennel seed, and mint.

Bring to a boil and continue boiling until the color of the water changes to a warm brown.

Strain out the seeds and mint leaves.

Add lemon juice and sweetener to taste.

Enjoy a cup of this tea after meals. It will help to reduce burping, gas, and abdominal discomfort from bloating.

CHAPTER SEVEN

IMPLEMENTING FOOD IMMUNOTHERAPY

Before we dive into the big picture of how desensitization is performed, it's important to understand what's going on at a molecular level. So let's have a mini immunology lesson, shall we? It can be helpful to think about immunotherapy for food allergens as occurring in four "steps," starting from initial exposure to the food and culminating in the production of protective "blocking" antibody instead of allergic IgE antibody. Let's walk through these steps below.

Step One: Allergen Introduction. The most straight-forward step. The food allergen is simply introduced into the body, in our case either sublingually (drops under the tongue) or orally (ingesting by mouth).

Step Two: Antigen Processing. This second step hinges on the efforts of antigen-presenting cells (APCs), the scavenger cells of the immune system. Their job is to circulate in your skin, respiratory tissues, and GI mucosa (the wet skin lining your digestive tract) and continuously sample the environment through phagocytosis. Phago-cytosis is a process by which the APC captures material and pulls it into itself for processing (much like eating something, albeit on a teeny tiny scale). APCs indiscrimi-nately gobble up what they find and rapidly travel to local lymph nodes. For example, if these APCs encounter an antigen in your mouth, they will travel to the lymph nodes under your jaw and neck. If they encounter the antigen in your gut, they will go to the mesenteric lymph nodes, or those that reside alongside your intestines. While the APCs travel to the lymph nodes, they stop sampling the environment and shift their focus to breaking down the already-captured allergen protein into small fragments called peptides.

Step Three: Antigen Presentation and Treg **Stimulation.** Once in the lymph nodes, the APCs earn their name and "present" the peptide antigens to T lymphocytes (a type of white blood cell) in the lymph tissue. Imagine the APCs ceremoniously removing the peptide antigens from their pockets and proudly announcing, "Here, look what I found!" Receptors on the surface of the T cells recognize these peptides. This interaction between T cell and APC enhances the activity of regulatory T cells of the immune system, or Tregs. Tregs promote immunologic tolerance, are anti-inflammatory, and produce cell-signaling molecules called cytokines. Two of the most important cytokines involved in desensitization are interleukin 10 (IL-10) and transforming growth factor beta (TGF beta). These are produced in large quantities when regulatory T cells are activated.

Step Four: Anergic Response. When other white blood cells and immune cells are exposed to the food allergen in the presence of IL-10 and TGF beta, it stimulates the following important changes in the immune system:

- Cells responsible for releasing histamine in the event of allergic reactions, such as mast cells and basophils, become *less* reactive. This means they will be less likely to degranulate, or burst open, and release histamine and other chemical mediators of allergic reactions upon future exposure to the food allergen.

- T cells decrease production of the proinflammatory cytokines that promote allergic symptoms, such as IL-4, IL-5, and IL-13. Instead, the T cells produce cytokines associated with what is called anergy, or a nonallergic response.

- B cells, the white blood cells that produce our antibodies, undergo a process called class switching. Each B cell is designated to produce a certain kind of antibody. Some B cells produce IgA, some produce IgG, and some produce IgE. During desensitization, B cells that originally produced IgE class switch and instead start producing IgG or IgA antibodies. The IgA and IgG are capable of binding to an allergenic protein before it even has the chance to bind to IgE antibodies. So, as the quantity of allergen-specific IgA and IgG goes up and the quantity of allergen-specific IgE goes down, the risk of an allergic reaction is reduced.

The cascade of these four steps is initiated each time the patient is exposed to precise quantities of the food allergen. It's a positive feedback loop: the more frequently the patient is exposed to the allergen, the more of these changes you will see. The next time our patient is exposed, she'll be able to handle just a little bit more, and that exposure will stimulate even more anti-inflammatory activity, and so on and so forth. Eventually, we'll have prompted enough anergy in the immune system to allow our patient to tolerate the ingestion of a *full* serving of the food—a dose that previously would have easily triggered anaphylaxis.

We must remind ourselves, however, that the safety of desensitization is predicated on the delivery of *very small doses* of allergen that increase incrementally over time. If one neglects this reality and introduces a large amount of allergen all at once, the patient is at an extremely high risk of experiencing a systemic reaction. Successful desensitization needs to strike the delicate balance between pushing the immune system's limits just enough but not too far. This is yet another reason to ensure that any food allergen desensitization is performed only under the supervision of a board-certified allergist and immunologist. Remember, we are trying to save kids, not hurt them. So no corner-cutting allowed!

CHARLIE'S GAME PLAN

Remember Charlie, our Chicago Cubs fan who was recently in my office for his graduation day? Before his treatment, he struggled with a severe peanut allergy and history of anaphylaxis to even small amounts of peanut ingestion. One tiny accidental bite of a cookie landed him in the ER and earned him a shot of epinephrine.

With patience and commitment to his treatment program, Charlie graduated from peanut OIT and was able to attend his much-anticipated baseball game. The road to home plate wasn't easy, though. At the onset of his treatment, Charlie's parents were understandably apprehensive about my ability to ensure their son wouldn't experience the severe reactions he'd had in the past—a fear compounded by bloodwork indicating a high ratio of peanut sIgE to total IgE.

I reassured them that my plan was designed to respect the sensitivity of Charlie's immune system and that we would begin treatment with an extremely low dose of peanut protein. Because Charlie had a high sIgE/total

IgE ratio and a history of severe anaphylaxis with even small amounts of exposure, I decided to prep his immune system for OIT with a lead-in therapy of SLIT. This type of immunotherapy involves giving the patient increasing doses of allergenic food extract via drops administered under the surface of the tongue.

SLIT: A BRIDGE TO OIT

In Charlie's case, I designed a six-month-long course of SLIT beginning with a single drop of a highly diluted preparation of peanut extract. This dose had the protein equivalent of only 1/1,000,000 of a peanut! (Knowing this made his mom feel *much* better.) Charlie held this single drop under his tongue for two minutes, giving the antigen-presenting cells—those scavenger cells in the tissues of his mouth—enough time to travel to the drop, gobble up the allergen, and take it to the lymph nodes under his jaw. After two minutes, he swallowed his accumulated saliva and took a sip of water, swished it in his mouth, and drank more water. Then we watched him in the office for thirty minutes before sending him home.

Why the observation period? We're aware that symptoms can occur anytime you introduce a food allergen back into the body. There is always a small, but real, risk of triggering an allergic reaction. Patients undergoing SLIT may experience some transient itching in the mouth or throat. It's unlikely with the first low-concentration dose, but it is a relatively common side effect as doses are ramped up. This is not a cause for concern—it's simply evidence that the immune system has recognized the allergen. However, we want to ensure that any symptoms that do occur after dosing are mild and self-limited. Also, because this is the first time the patient's immune system is "seeing" this dose deliberately, we want to make sure that the dose isn't too much for the patient to handle. It is incredibly rare to experience a serious reaction after SLIT, but I can guarantee that if a significant reaction does occur, you would much rather be in my office than in your car! The observation period is so important because it helps confirm to the parent, the patient, and to our medical providers that the dose was well tolerated.

After we confirmed that Charlie's sublingual dose was indeed well tolerated, I instructed Charlie's parents to give him that same dose every day for the next week. Then I scheduled Charlie to return to my office the following week for an increased dose from the same concentration of peanut SLIT. Instead of one drop, he received two drops. The week after that, three drops. Then four drops. Next, we transitioned to a stronger concentration of SLIT drops and once again ramped up on the number of drops within that bottle. Over the course of six months, Charlie went from a highly diluted preparation—the equivalent, remember, of 1/1,000,000 of a peanut—to a final dose equivalent to 1/250 of a peanut.

As you can see, SLIT is a long process with conservative dosing targets. At times, it can feel excruciatingly slow. However, in the properly selected patient, SLIT can mean the difference between sailing through food allergen desensitization and having a rocky road. In my experience, most patients who complete a preliminary round of SLIT enjoy a very smooth course of treatment when they start OIT. Bloodwork performed after six months of SLIT also consistently demonstrates an increase in allergen-specific IgG4 (recall that this is one of the protective antibodies produced in step four of desensitization). I have developed my own SLIT protocols for eggs, milk, peanuts, tree nuts, seafood, and seeds. I have refined these protocols and the selection criteria for food SLIT over the years to improve tolerability of the regimen and to help capture more of the patients who might benefit from this hybrid protocol. It is important to emphasize here that the use of SLIT as a lead-in to OIT is not de rigueur in all practices, but it is steadily gaining traction as evidence of SLIT's utility grows.

REDUCING RISK

As mentioned above, the risk of allergic reactions in the sublingual phase is relatively low due to the small doses of allergenic protein being administered. Generally, any symptoms we observe during SLIT are local and self-limited, typically involving itching in the mouth. In fact, it's standard to experience mild transient itching for the first two or three days of a particular dose. Most of the itching we see with SLIT resolves within five minutes of drinking water. If a patient reports consistently experiencing itching lasting fifteen or twenty minutes after a dose, I am unlikely to increase his dose the following week. "I think you need longer on this dose," I'll tell him. "Your body is not ready to go to the next dose yet. I want to see only transient symptoms, or no symptoms at all, before I'm ready to updose you."

While uncommon, there are other risks associated with sublingual therapy, and it's important to be aware of how these reactions might present so we can employ strategies to prevent them from happening. If a patient has eczema or very chapped lips, for example, allergens can gain access to the immune system through that compromised skin barrier. For this reason, significant swelling can occur if SLIT drops make contact with dry, chafed lips. To mitigate this risk, I encourage my patients to apply lip balm liberally and to refrain from licking their lips. If there is any perioral dermatitis or facial eczema, I also treat this with simple emollients or anti-inflammatory medication to heal the skin before dosing. Allergens from immunotherapy solution can also gain direct access to the bloodstream through exposed capillary vessels in a canker sore or in the bed of a lost tooth. This may trigger a serious reaction. Therefore, we avoid dosing directly onto compromised mucosa to reduce the chances of an unexpected reaction.

Remember, low risk doesn't mean no risk! It's essential to keep safety first and foremost in our minds and take every necessary precaution to safeguard patients during desensitization.

RAPID DESENSITIZATION

Once Charlie completed his peanut SLIT protocol—which, remember, is not needed for all patients—he was ready to transition into OIT. OIT begins with *rapid desensitization*. Rapid desensitization is a procedure during which an allergen is introduced into the body as increasing doses given at frequent intervals over the course of hours to days. Essentially, the allergen is "sprinkled in" over a set period rather than introduced as a "downpour" all at once. This prepares the body to accept allergen introduction safely.

The key to understanding why rapid desensitization works is to first comprehend how allergic reactions are triggered. Classic type I hypersensitivity reactions are precipitated by IgE antibody interactions on the surface of mast cells. IgE antibodies are in the shape of a capital letter Y. The trunk of the Y is the part that fits into the receptor on the surface of the mast cell, and the arms of the Y have binding sites on the end of them that are specific for a particular protein allergen. Cross-linking of IgE occurs when two or more mast-cell-bound IgE antibodies link up to the same allergen. (It's almost like holding hands.) Cross-linking prompts the mast cell to burst open and release histamine, leukotrienes, and cytokines into the surrounding tissue. This process is called degranulation, and it is the critical event in a cascade of both early- and late-phase inflammation that occurs during an allergic reaction. Our goal is to prevent mast cell degranulation. No degranulation equals no allergic reaction.

How do we prevent degranulation? Prevent cross-linking! Remember, cross-linking of IgE requires that at least two separate IgE antibody molecules bind to the *same unit* of allergenic protein. This can only occur if those binding sites on the IgE are not already occupied. Cross-linking occurs rapidly when a substantial dose of allergen is introduced into the body all at once because there are simultaneously high concentrations of both allergen and allergen-binding sites. However, rapid desensitization avoids this scenario. At the beginning of a rapid desensitization, there are a high number of available allergen-binding sites but a low concentration of allergen. That means large-scale cross-linking does not occur. As the introduction of allergen is spread out over the course of multiple hours, most of the available antigen-binding sites gradually become bound with their own allergen, leaving no room for shared binding or opportunity to cross-link. The rapid desensitization procedure ends with a relatively high concentration of allergen in the body but very few open allergen-binding sites available for them. Therefore, the rapid desensitization process manipulates the balance of allergen and binding sites to prevent massive degranulation. It dramatically reduces the risk of experiencing a systemic allergic reaction.

During Charlie's rapid desensitization to peanut, he received doses every fifteen minutes from increasing concentrations of peanut flour suspension. The first dose was incredibly small—only 1/200,000 of a peanut. After each dose, we observed him to be sure he tolerated it well, and then we offered another dose. Over the course of the day, Charlie had more than twenty doses and ultimately built up to a final dose of approximately 1/100 of a peanut.

You may have noticed that the starting dose of rapid desensitization was substantially lower than Charlie's last dose of peanut SLIT—1/250 of a peanut. This is by design. In fact, the first three-fourths of Charlie's rapid desensitization consisted of doses he had seen before during SLIT. He built up a small level of tolerance with SLIT, breezed through the initial doses of rapid desensitization, and then went on to significantly surpass his final SLIT dose by 250 percent.

You might be wondering, what is the difference between sublingual desensitization and rapid desensitization if some of the doses are the same? Put simply, sublingual desensitization takes a long time to go from tiny amounts to slightly less tiny amounts. Rapid desensitization, on the other hand, moves from tiny amounts to visible amounts in six hours, not six months.

Rapid desensitization can understandably be a bit nerve-racking, so we try to distract from the anxiety with lots of movies, board games, and safe snacks. These distractions are also needed because when rapid desensitization goes as planned (almost always), it can get pretty tedious and routine. That's the way I like it! I always tell my patients with a wink and a smile, "If I ask you how rapid desensitization is going, and you tell me it's boring, I am doing a great job! I'll bring the boredom; you bring the fun." After the last dose of his rapid desensitization procedure, Charlie was observed for an additional hour to rule out any delayed reactions. I then sent him home with his final dose of peanut suspension to take at home daily until his next appointment, when we planned to challenge him with a slightly higher dose and continue the process of peanut desensitization.

OIT BUILDUP: THE STEPPING STONES TO GRADUATION

After rapid desensitization, Charlie moved into the buildup phase of OIT. OIT buildup included daily home-based dosing and periodic medically supervised dose increases, followed by a period of in-office observation. Dose after dose, moving ever closer to a full serving of peanut. The buildup phase is where most of the "OIT magic" happened, and we saw proof that Charlie's ability to tolerate peanut was steadily increasing over time. Charlie's OIT updosing continued for twelve months (but can take as little as six months in some patients). Each time Charlie came to the office, he was challenged with the next dose in his protocol.

Office visits during OIT aren't only limited to administering a new dose—they're also an opportunity to check in on the patient's overall health and confirm that food immunotherapy is proceeding without bothersome side effects. At each visit, patients are asked detailed questions about their dosing. I want to know if they've been taking the dose regularly, if they are experiencing any side effects or if there have been any health changes since the last visit. We ensure that rhinitis, asthma, and eczema are under control and that the patient isn't experiencing any GI issues. We also confirm that we have all medications and supplements listed in our records accurately.

It's essential to inquire specifically about each of the points above because pertinent health issues commonly go unnoticed or unreported when patients become accustomed to the routine of updose appointments. I have had many patients come in and say, "Yeah, I'm feeling good!" When I perform the physical exam, however, it paints a different picture. I must explain, "You say you're feeling good, but you're actually wheezing. Your asthma's flaring up, and I don't think you realized it. If we updosed you today, you might have a bad reaction. So let's change the focus of today's visit to getting your asthma under control, and we can resume your updose schedule once you feel better." Structuring our visits to address the whole patient ensures that we don't miss any changes to health that might impact the safety of dosing.

Once again, I cannot overemphasize the critical importance of adequate medical supervision during this process. **OIT is absolutely NOT something your family can take on by yourselves.** You might think, "It seems simple enough. I just need to do a little math and measure out some peanut flour." To this, I reply, "Patience, young grasshopper! What people need to understand is that the complexity of OIT isn't the protocol itself. Rather, the difficulty lies in the safe implementation of the protocol." During OIT, multiple health variables are constantly in flux and need to be deftly juggled. Attempting to navigate the process on your own is a potentially life-threatening mistake.

Charlie's OIT dose was initially the form of a liquid suspension, which was preservative-free and required refrigeration and replacement every two weeks. Updosing was continued with liquid until we reached a dose of approximately one-tenth of a peanut. Charlie then transitioned to capsules that contained a precisely measured dose of defatted peanut flour. This was a welcome convenience, as encapsulated OIT doses are shelf-stable and small enough to travel with easily. But these weren't the type of capsules you swallow. Instead, the capsules were emptied into a food vehicle, such as pudding, applesauce, oatmeal, or yogurt. Some creative families even incorporate the flour dose into homemade chocolates or marinara sauce. Encapsulated peanut flour doses were continued until reaching the equivalent of one half of a peanut.

The capsule phase of peanut OIT transitions directly into eating actual roasted peanuts. As you can imagine, this can seem surreal after a lifetime of avoidance. So many parents describe a sense of trepidation mixed with amazement as they walk into the grocery store and pick up their first tin of the extra-large Virginia peanuts we recommend for dosing. I've even had a few selfies texted to me from the nut aisle! Charlie started by eating half a peanut kernel once daily. We continued to increase the daily dose until he was eating twelve peanuts a day. Charlie continued ingesting twelve peanuts daily for a month and then returned to my office for his twenty-four-peanut challenge.

Some patients and families are understandably nervous when they learn we are going straight from twelve to twenty-four peanuts. "It's is an enormous jump! How can we do that safely?" they ask. I remind them of the dose-dependent nature of anergy induction: "The more you eat, the better it works." By the time we reached the twenty-four-peanut challenge, the desensitization and anergy induction weren't just beginning; they were already in full swing. We felt confident that Charlie had built up the ability to tolerate a full serving of peanut containing six grams of peanut protein. The truth is, the risk of reacting during a twenty-four-peanut challenge is probably lower than it is in the early phases of immunotherapy when the individual doses are small, but desensitization is not yet firmly established.

MANAGING SIDE EFFECTS AND REACTIONS

Just as in SLIT, side effects and reactions can occur during OIT. It's important to have clear protocols on how to manage these issues, so we are prepared to quickly implement them should side effects appear.

Mild reactions during OIT are not uncommon and tend to be self-limited. Transient itching of the mouth and throat can occur, but generally resolve within a few minutes without medication. In these cases, I recommend rinsing the mouth, drinking water, and eating safe foods which are moisture-rich (such as applesauce).

Abdominal pain, gas, reflux, nausea, and vomiting have also occurred, and are among the most common side effects of treatment. These symptoms are typically managed with the following: dietary modification, anti-reflux medication, and immunotherapy dosing adjustments. The vast majority of patients are able to resolve these symptoms with the above measures and complete the immunotherapy protocols.

Although it is not common, when the above measures are insufficient to control gastrointestinal symptoms during OIT, one must consider the possibility of eosinophilic esophagitis. Eosinophilic esophagitis is an inflammatory condition of the lining of the esophagus (food pipe) which can be worsened by exposure to environmental or ingested allergens. Symptoms include trouble swallowing, a sensation of food getting stuck in the throat, and severe reflux symptoms that do not respond to standard antacid medication. EoE is diagnosed by endoscopy (a procedure involving inserting a small camera into the digestive tract through the mouth) and biopsy which demonstrates an accumulation of eosinophils (allergic white blood cells) in the lining of the esophagus.

New research suggests that there is a genetic basis for eosinophilic esophagitis. Therefore, it is believed that symptoms of EoE that develop in patients undergoing OIT represent an "unmasking" of the disease process in genetically susceptible individuals who were otherwise asymptomatic due to allergen avoidance. When therapy is discontinued and strict elimination of the allergen re-instituted, EoE symptoms generally resolve within a few months. In most cases, active EoE is a legitimate reason to discontinue OIT. However, there may be an alternate solution that enables continuation of treatment in select cases.

Some centers have identified a syndrome of delayed vomiting and GI symptoms (two-to-six hours after dosing), which is associated with an increase in the blood eosinophil count. This syndrome has been termed ELORS (Eosinophilic Esophagitis Like Oral Immunotherapy Related Syndrome). It is possible to continue to treat patients with ELORS with OIT, by reducing the dose to a very low level and maintaining the low dose for months at a time before attempting increases.

Any time that a food allergen is deliberately administered to an allergic individual, the potential for a body-wide allergic reaction (anaphylaxis) exists. Although it is not typical, anaphylaxis has occurred in the context of oral immunotherapy dosing. When systemic reactions are noted, they are immediately treated with epinephrine and additional adjunctive medications as appropriate. Systemic reactions do not preclude the patient from moving forward with the protocol. In fact, most patients who have required epinephrine in the course of treatment go on to graduate from their respective desensitization programs.

TREATMENT MILESTONES

When a patient is pursuing a lengthy treatment protocol such as OIT, it can sometimes feel as though the end will never be in sight. Therefore, we make a point of benchmarking and celebrating small victories. Dosing milestones are an important part of the OIT process because they provide reassurance of progress made and give patients and families something to look forward to—this is especially important for young children. When patients begin OIT, I map out the trajectory of treatment in advance and identify certain doses that carry special significance. Below are a few of the milestones we highlight during peanut OIT, but other foods have their own milestone doses as well. (Note: These milestones are fairly conservative and err on the side of caution and safety.)

THREE PEANUTS

Many patients with food allergies avoid not only foods containing their allergen but also avoid foods processed on shared equipment or in shared facilities. This can be incredibly disruptive to quality of life because it limits so many foods from the diet. My practice is to encourage patients to continue consuming foods that have been well tolerated, even if labeled for cross-contamination. However, the worry of a possible reaction to cross-contamination often looms large.

When a patient pursuing peanut OIT reaches the three-peanut mark, I clear them to consume items labeled for cross-contamination as well as foods cooked in peanut oil. (Although highly refined peanut oil is typically safe for peanut-allergic patients, many patients choose to avoid it out of an abundance of caution.) I'll tell them, "You're all good. Go ahead and enjoy those cakes and cookies you've been avoiding. You're going to be fine. If you can eat three peanuts safely, you can definitely eat something that may have trace amounts of peanut protein in it." It always puts a smile on my face when my patients text me pictures of themselves eating their first doughnut, a fried chicken sandwich, or a cupcake with other kids at a birthday party. These seemingly little things are huge to a kid who has never been able to enjoy such freedoms before.

EIGHT PEANUTS

Some patients dislike the taste of peanuts enough that they have no desire to eat any peanut items outside of their daily dose. These patients aren't interested in peanut butter, Snickers bars, or Thai food. They just want the confidence of being protected from an accidental ingestion. These patients are always excited to reach the eight-peanut dose, which is the daily maintenance dose in the peanut OIT protocol our office follows and is high enough to protect our patients from the risks of accidental peanut ingestion. I tell them, "If you can eat eight peanuts every day and maintain that dose, you don't need to worry about having a bad reaction to a bite of a peanut butter cookie or Kung Pao chicken."

Many patients, however, *do* want to freely eat Asian foods, peanut butter cups, or other peanut-containing foods. For these patients, I encourage them to pursue a twenty-four-peanut challenge. This challenge proves that the patient can tolerate a substantial dose of peanut protein, which is unlikely to be exceeded in a typical meal even when peanuts are a known ingredient. This milestone offers a new layer of culinary freedom, enabling patients to live life without reading labels.

An important caveat: Even in the maintenance phase of immunotherapy, exercise restrictions must still be followed after deliberate food allergen ingestion. Otherwise, the patient risks triggering a reaction. In fact, all of our safety rules still apply after graduation. If a graduate eats a peanut butter and jelly sandwich, for example, she can't jump on a trampoline right afterward. Completing a desensitization protocol doesn't mean the allergy is gone. Rather, it means the food allergy has been effectively managed. Remember, food allergen desensitization is a fix, not a cure. Overall, though, the amount of freedom and degree of safety we're able to introduce via OIT is a game changer.

After graduation, I remind my patients that we've got a good "fix" in place but to keep in mind that future adjustments can always be made. Because regular exposure of the immune system to the allergen is the best way to maintain desensitization and induce anergy, most patients choose to continue daily dosing after graduation. However, I do have some patients who have experienced such a dramatic immune response to eating their allergen every day that the ratio of food-specific IgE:IgG4 has dropped precipitously after a few years. I offer these patients the option to reduce their dosing to two to three times a week. Some of my colleagues have even offered their patients the opportunity to hold dosing for a month or more and then pursue an in-office oral challenge to assess for the ability to maintain sustained immunotolerance without regular dosing.

ADDRESSING MULTIPLE ALLERGIES

In chapter 5, I briefly touched on how to address multiple food allergies when planning food desensitization therapy. Now, let's delve a little deeper into treatment options for those patients dealing with more than one food allergy. There are three approaches I take when determining how to organize an immunotherapy schedule:

- **Option 1:** We can start by attacking the food allergy that is most impactful to the patient's quality of life. Sometimes patients and their families will report that a nut allergy feels manageable due to improved awareness, but another coexisting allergy is poorly understood and more difficult to live with. Parents may say, "There are so many places and products that are peanut-free and tree nut-free that we feel comfortable with that allergy for now, but the milk allergy is hard for us. It makes it difficult for my child to feel included or for us to be able to go anywhere that feels safe. If we could just handle this milk allergy first, we think our lives would be so much better." In this case, the decision is clear. We start with milk.

- **Option 2:** We can take advantage of food allergen cross-reactivity profiles. Sometimes a patient with a high concentration of peanut-specific IgE will have lower concentrations of IgE to foods that may share some cross-reactive proteins with peanut (e.g., hazelnut, almond, and soy). The patient may still have a history of reacting to these foods, so they must be avoided. Families inquire whether it would be most prudent to begin with the food allergens with lower IgE values and then work up to peanut. However, I usually opt for the opposite approach. I like to address the big, bad food allergy first. A successful peanut desensitization may also desensitize for cross-reactive proteins the peanut shares with tree nuts and legumes. That means there is a good chance that after peanut OIT, the patient may be able to proceed directly to oral challenges for the remaining food allergens. This approach saves patients the time, effort, and expense of needing multiple rounds of OIT.

- **Option 3:** Sometimes it is practical to treat multiple food allergies at once. For example, I have successfully treated multiple tree nuts simultaneously and have also designed combination protocols for peanut, tree nuts, and seeds. However, research centers such as Stanford are actively researching ways to desensitize *all* the major food allergens simultaneously. To accomplish this safely and quickly requires premedication with anti-IgE medication called omalizumab (FDA-approved for severe asthma and chronic hives). Injecting patients with omalizumab prior to the initiation of OIT binds up free-floating IgE, preventing it from attaching to the receptors on the surface of the mast cell. This helps protect against allergic reactions and allows patients to tolerate certain combinations of allergens that they might not have been able to previously. The omalizumab does not need to be continued indefinitely and can typically be discontinued after graduation.

The major benefit of using omalizumab is that it enables patients to complete multifood immunotherapy quickly. But how important is it to complete OIT quickly? It depends on the situation. For some patients, timing matters, especially if they will soon be leaving home for college. I have used omalizumab as an adjunctive therapy for select patients, but my personal preference is to perform immunotherapy for foods without the crutch of additional medication. Why? Some of the omalizumab study participants have done well initially but, once weaned off the omalizumab, have started reacting to their food allergen doses. Instead of using omalizumab as a short-term assist, I would rather take a slower and more integrative approach to definitively manage whatever allergic inflammation I can on the front end. I can do this by utilizing aeroallergen immunotherapy, performing SLIT to gradually stimulate the anergic response in the immune system, or any number of the other approaches outlined in previous chapters. However, I still keep omalizumab in my arsenal, especially for patients with severe asthma that is difficult to bring under control.

WHAT HAPPENS AFTER GRADUATION?

Similar to graduating from school in a cap and gown, graduation from an OIT treatment program is a time of celebration and an opportunity to relax after putting in months and years of hard work. The days, weeks, and years after graduation, however, still require effort in the form of consistent maintenance doses and continued observation of safety precautions. Thankfully, there is a bit of wiggle room.

Sometimes, for patients who have been in the maintenance phase for a long time without experiencing any reactions, I'll broach the idea of decreasing the exercise restriction from two hours to a shorter time. This helps with the convenience of fitting dosing into their routines and activities, especially as kids grow older. I would not eliminate the exercise restriction altogether, however, unless a patient opted to undergo an exercise challenge in the office postmaintenance dose—an option that none of my patients have been keen to pursue.

Missing your dose once in a while is entirely acceptable in the maintenance phase. In fact, there are some situations in which I tell people to just skip their dose altogether. I like to use the example of an amusement park to illustrate this point to my patients and their families. Say you didn't dose in the morning because you knew you needed to make it to the park on time and hit the rides. It's a hot summer day. You're in the sun and eating junk food. You are probably not drinking as much water as you should. You've been running around for hours, and by the time you leave, it's 10:00 p.m. You are overheated and exhausted, and then you realize you haven't dosed yet. Should you dose at 11:00 p.m. and hope for the best? No! In situations like this, I *implore* my patients to skip the dose that day. There is too much risk of reaction. Better safe than sorry.

For this reason, I tell people if they want the flexibility to skip on days like I described above, it's incredibly important they don't skip on the other days. Whenever it's practical, they should aim to take their prescribed dose every day because it gives them the flexibility they may need on other days when it is not possible to dose.

For example, I had a patient who had already been in maintenance for peanuts for three years and had been taking his dose very consistently, every day. He was accepted to a weeklong summer camp in the north woods of Michigan, with very little cell phone signal, no easy access to major roads, and no hospitals or emergency medical facilities close by. His mother asked what I thought about holding off on dosing while he was away. Taking into consideration the consistency of his dosing over the previous three years and how well he had done, I permitted him to skip dosing while he was at camp. When he got back home, he took a slightly lower dose for a couple of days and then a three-fourths of a dose. Within a week of returning home from camp, he had resumed his full maintenance dose. Didn't miss a beat!

This scenario is early evidence of sustained immunotolerance. The ideal result after completing food allergen desensitization is that protection from reactions be maintained even in the absence of formal dosing. The goal is for periodic incorporation into the diet (eating like a nonallergic person) to be sufficient. Notice that I don't say that the food need not be ingested at all. It is never a good idea to go back to strict avoidance after OIT because the protection gained during immunotherapy can be lost. The hope is that over time, we'll be able to identify biomarkers to help determine who is more likely to develop sustained immunotolerance and who truly needs to dose in a more regimented fashion. I think that is where the ratio of IgE to the IgG4 comes into play. I like to see the food-specific IgE:IgG4 ratio go as low as possible, as these are the patients most likely to do well with intermittent dosing.

Now that Charlie has graduated from peanut immuno-therapy, he doesn't just sail off into the sunset. He will still see me in clinic a couple of times a year because health maintenance is part of OIT maintenance. We will mon-itor his progress with OIT, his overall health, as well as his yearly lab values. With consistency and dedication to following his treatment plan, Charlie may also one day receive the happy news that frequency of dosing and dose-related exercise restrictions can be relaxed. After all, that's the goal of food allergen desensitization. To make life safer. Easier. Better.

CONCLUSION

Desensitization therapies for food allergy continue to evolve at a rapid clip. The approach to precision medicine for food allergen desensitization I've described extensively in this book also looks a little different for each patient and is implemented differently by each allergist. As a relatively new therapy, food allergen desensitization is a practice in motion, and change is inevitable. My colleagues and I continue to modify and refine these protocols as we gain more experience and feedback from our patients. In fact, it is likely that by the time you're reading this book, we may have already enhanced and modified some of the ways in which we deliver treatment for food allergies. This is a good thing! We want physicians in clinical practice and researchers to continue evaluating the safety and efficacy of existing protocols, identifying areas for optimization, and improving current practice.

After all, stagnation equals deterioration. If there are safer or more efficient ways in which to deliver care, we want to ensure our treatments consistently evolve to apply the new evidence.

What I've detailed in this book is *my* philosophical approach to food desensitization, but by no stretch of the imagination do I mean to imply that this is the *only* way to implement the therapy. What you've read about here is a guide and an outline for understanding how this process works, why you may wish to consider it as an option, and how to take a "whole-person" view of health in the context of desensitization. Again, the information presented here isn't a prescription, and it most definitely is *not* meant to serve as an instruction manual. The best interest of our patients necessitates that a certified allergist evaluate each patient, determine the best course of therapy for that unique individual, and implement the prescribed treatment under scrupulous medical supervision.

GUIDANCE TO PATIENTS AND FAMILIES

If you're a parent who is wondering how best to advocate for your child with food allergies and trying to decide if pursuing a treatment for the food allergy is the right choice, I offer this guidance:

· **Keep meticulous records.** I cannot emphasize

enough how helpful this step is to an allergist when meeting a new patient. Having access to detailed records of health in early childhood, reaction history, treatment history, and trends over time helps us personalize our approaches and mitigate risk factors that we identify in our patient's history. However, a gigantic binder with copies of every office visit or urgent care summary is too much to sift through and can be overwhelming. Instead, whittle the records down to the bare essentials and incorporate it all into a single digital document. I recommend that families create an Excel or Google spreadsheet with separate sheets within the document for medical conditions, reaction history, test results, and medications. Update this spreadsheet whenever your child has a new medical diagnosis, a medication change, new testing results, or experiences a reaction. Print a hard copy before your office visits to give to the doctor. Having this consolidated data at the ready will save you valuable time during your office visits, and your physicians will be so pleased that they will want to hug you with gratitude. You can find a template of this spreadsheet at www.foodallergyfix.com.

· **Learn as much as you can.** The initial impulse of any parent whose child receives a medical diagnosis is to immediately go online and devour as much information about the condition as possible. You know what they say: "A food allergy parent does better research than the FBI!" I encourage families to heed this instinct, but I also recognize that the internet is full of inaccurate and sensationalized information. Therefore, I steer families toward vetted resources that will offer accurate information. The national (American Academy of Allergy, Asthma & Immunology; American College of Allergy, Asthma, and Immunology) and international (World Allergy Organization) allergy societies, Centers for Disease Control and Prevention, National Institutes of Health, and food allergy advocacy organizations are great places to start for general food allergy information. For food treatment-related information and support from other families who have walked in your shoes, there are a number of focused Facebook groups that many patients find to be an invaluable resource for support and experience. A number of patients who have completed OIT or participated in clinical trials have kept blogs and written books to document their treatment journeys. Go ahead, read and digest it all! Then ask your trusted allergists for their opinions on the data you have collected in your readings. After all, these *are* the people who have invested their entire careers into understanding how the immune system works. They often have insights you may not have considered. Now, you may be fearful of discussing your desire to consider food allergen desensitization, worried that they will belittle you or simply dismiss you from their practice.

Don't be scared, and don't feel like you need to keep your hope of a treatment a secret. Your relationship with your family allergist should be collaborative, not adversarial, and any allergist worth their salt will at least listen to you and be willing to learn more. You can help make the discussion with your doctor a productive one by educating yourself beforehand. When you understand the treatments available, you'll be better prepared to meaningfully discuss your options with your allergist and immunologist.

- **Get your foot in the door.** If you do decide that you want to pursue the option of meeting with an OIT allergist to determine if your child is a candidate for desensitization, great! Meeting with the allergist for a consultation doesn't mean you have to start right away, but establishing care at a practice experienced in the treatment you are considering is a good idea. This is especially true because the ratio of providers who are able to offer this therapy to the number of patients interested in the therapy is very low. Due to this imbalance, many offices have waiting lists. So even if you're on the fence, it's to your benefit to meet with an allergist to establish a relationship, get your questions answered, and if needed, get onto the wait list. There is some evidence that immunotherapy works especially well in younger immune systems, so it's fine to meet with an allergist even if you believe your child isn't old enough to pursue OIT yet. Tip:

Once you have decided that desensitization is the right choice for your family, any wait can seem like an eternity. Please be patient with the office staff helping you schedule your appointment. They are here to help you and may be in the unenviable position of informing you and hundreds of other anxious food allergy parents that due to the demand for desensitization therapy, the initial consultation appointment won't be available for months. Be *kind* in the face of this frustration. You catch more flies with honey.

THE TIME IS NOW

Just like any medical treatment, food allergen desensitization isn't right for everyone. However, if your child has a potentially life-threatening food allergy that significantly limits quality of life, the process can be transformative. From a safety standpoint, successfully completing OIT significantly reduces the risk of experiencing anaphylaxis from accidental ingestion of a food allergen. This is the primary goal, obviously. But what really triggers "all the feels" for families is the impact of food allergen desensitization on the emotional well-being of patients. Parents remember all the times their children were left out and couldn't be "normal" kids. They think about the times kids came home from trick or treating and almost all their candy had to be given away. They recall how invitations to birthday parties gradually trickled to a halt because other parents didn't know how to manage food allergies or keep their children safe. They recount stories of classroom desks being moved to a corner during holiday parties because somebody brought in a food containing an allergen. In these circumstances, children with food allergies were, in effect, punished while everyone else celebrated. These are the situations parents remember. These are the situations children remember. All this speaks to one of the real beauties of this therapy: it enables inclusivity. Desensitization helps kids with food allergy feel like regular kids again.

I'm not suggesting that SLIT and OIT are the only options for children with food allergies. Epicutaneous immunotherapy, Chinese herbal therapy, peptide immunotherapy, and augmented DNA vaccines have all shown varying degrees of promise. Researchers put blood, sweat, money, and tears into advocating for children, and I firmly believe we should continue researching any therapy that might help patients overcome food allergies. The rapid expansion of research into potential food allergy treatments is cause for optimism and gratitude. I do envision a future where we can combine these therapies to optimize results. However, at this time, oral desensitization is the most accessible and cost-effective treatment, and the only one providing such robust protection against reactions. As we continue to refine our protocols, OIT will become even safer and better tolerated. What we need is for every population center to have at least a handful of allergists skilled in food allergen desensitization so families don't need to travel long distances or wait for years before gaining access to lifesaving therapy for their children. In my own conversations with colleagues, it is clear that there is a growing tide of qualified allergists sincerely interested in offering food allergen immunotherapy to their patients. My hope is that this book can give my colleagues the confidence to start implementing OIT in their practices and play at least a small role in increasing access to care for all of our patients.

There are those who argue that OIT is imperfect and that we should be holding out for a treatment that is more refined and standardized. I understand their desire to avoid risk for patients and to "do no harm." I really do. And given the current pace of medical advancements, it is altogether possible that twenty years from now, OIT will simply be the distant memory of a "quaint" medical procedure allergists utilized before a definitive cure for food allergies was available. Knowing this, why not just wait for the perfect treatment, and save ourselves the effort and risk that food allergen desensitization entails? Because we simply don't have the luxury of waiting! Each year, people are experiencing life-threatening reactions and dying, not because they contracted a severe infection or had rapidly progressive cancer or were involved in a major automobile accident but rather because they ate food. Let that sink in for a minute. *They died because they ate food.* Why are we content to live in a world where so many are afraid to feed our children?

So until there's a cure, there's OIT. I may not yet have the ability to *cure* food allergies, but what I do have is the power to *heal*. And I am losing patience with the voices telling me, my colleagues, and my patients that we just need to wait a little bit longer. I am a board-certified allergist with extensive training in the mechanisms and function of the immune system. I have specialized expertise in pediatric food allergies and years of experience in preventing and managing anaphylaxis. So guess what? I'm not waiting another five to ten years for a one-size-fits-all pill, patch, or injection. *Because my patients are each unique, and I already have the skills to design a precisely tailored treatment plan for each of them.* I don't need to hold out for an idiotproof protocol *because I'm no idiot.* Now, before one gets the wrong impression, let me be perfectly clear: I do not consider myself any special prodigy in the allergy world. Thousands of my colleagues around the globe have the same education and skillset that I do, and we can heal our patients *now*. We can own our expertise and use our skills to offer children safety and inclusion instead of fear and isolation. Or we can wait. In that time, how many patients will be told that "there are no treatments available"? Despite their best efforts at avoidance, how many of these patients will succumb to accidental ingestion?

Is it even ethical for us to withhold information about a viable treatment strategy when we know one exists?

I know firsthand that food allergen immunotherapy is time-consuming, emotionally exhausting, and potentially risky work—on the part of health professionals, patients, and their loved ones. But I can also attest that it is freeing, lifesaving, supremely gratifying work.

The Food Allergy Fix is work that needs doing.

Just ask Charlie.

FURTHER READING AND RESOURCES

(Descriptions come from websites and groups themselves.)

FOR PATIENTS AND FAMILIES

WEBSITES

- **Food Allergy Fix:** foodallergyfix.com. The companion website to this book. Educational videos, articles, and files to support you on your food allergen desensitization journey.
- **Kaneland Allergy & Asthma Center:** kanelandallergy.com. Dr. Bajowala's private allergy and immunology practice in North Aurora, Illinois.
- **Kaneland Food Allergy Foundation:** kfaf.org. The mission of the Kaneland Food Allergy Foundation is

to improve awareness of and access to evidence-based and life-changing treatment for patients with food allergy through educational initiatives, community outreach, and financial assistance.

- **OIT 101**: oit101.org. This website contains biographies and contact information for a number of board-certified allergists and immunologists offering OIT for food allergies. It also has links to published studies and research on the topic of food allergen desensitization, along with an FAQ.

FACEBOOK GROUPS AND PAGES

- **OIT 101**: facebook.com/groups/OIT101/. OIT 101 is the place to learn about food allergy desensitization offered by private-practice board-certified allergists.
- **Private Practice OIT:** facebook.com/groups/PrivatePracticeOIT/. Private Practice OIT supports people and families in food allergy desensitization offered by private practice board-certified allergists.

The above groups advocate OIT as a proven "safe and effective" treatment for food allergy/anaphylaxis to date. Their purpose is to unite you with a private board-certified allergist who may be able to help your child. It's their way of giving back after miraculous success with OIT treatment.

- **SLIT Support for Food Allergies:**
  facebook.com/groups/slitsupport/. This group allows
  members to share experiences, vent, rejoice, and help
  each other along the specific road of using SLIT for
  food allergies. The food allergy life can be tough, and
  the group offers each other emotional support. This
  group is *not* here to offer medical advice. A space that
  is safe for sharing is the number-one goal.
- **Food Allergy Treatment Talk (FATT):**
  facebook.com/groups/foodallergytreatmenttalk/.
  With a growing menu of current treatments from
  which to choose (and many more on the horizon),
  this page serves as a one-stop shop for sharing and
  discussing evidence-based scientific research related
  to improving—and one day, hopefully, eliminating—
  IgE-mediated food allergies (unrelated to intolerances/
  sensitivities) in people of all ages. Get the skinny at
  FATT!

FOR ALLERGISTS

- **FAST: Food Allergy Support Team:**
  facebook.com/foodallergysupportteam/. The purpose
  of Food Allergy Support Team is to improve the lives
  of people living with food allergies and their families
  by advancing the knowledge of food allergy prevention and treatment by enhancing the access to expert
  allergy care. This physician-led organization holds

regular meetings and a yearly educational conference. FAST has worked to develop an online registry to combine data from multiple practices offering food allergen desensitization into a single source.

- **OIT Society:** oitsociety.org/. This website is specifically for doctors. Doctors want to know how OIT works, if they should refer patients to OIT specialists, and how they can become an OIT provider. This group is here to help you serve the medical and food allergy communities.

ACKNOWLEDGMENTS

With God, all things are possible.

Mummy and Daddy (Maleka & Yusuf Shikari). Thank you for all the sacrifices you made so I could pursue my passion. From grade-school science projects to private-school tuition to helping me raise my babies—any credit and blessings accrued from my life's work rightfully flow back to you.

Mom and Dad (Nafisa and Yosef Bajowala). How blessed I am to have in-laws who treat me like their own daughter, always ready and able to support my professional and personal efforts with words of support and helping hands. Since joining your family, I have known nothing but love and kindness.

Mansoor. The doer to my dreamer. You are quite simply the reason that everything happens in my life. Thank you for being the driving force behind my writing this book, and for keeping me on task at every stage of the game. Thank you for convincing me to take time for fun, even when I felt I could never crawl out from under my mountain of work. Thank you for tolerating me when I was stressed, and for taking on extra duties at home or with the kids so I could focus. Thank you for silently handling all the tedious, but essential, logistics to get the Kaneland Food Allergy Foundation off the ground. Thank you for doing all this while traveling for your own job and juggling so many other projects. You are my most trusted advisor, the COO of my world, and my forever love.

Shehzad and Aqeel. Thank you for being the best kids a mom could ever wish for. Thank you for sharing me with thousands of sick children, since you were infants. There were so many times when I would leave before you woke and arrive home after you had fallen asleep, but still I received your unconditional love. You gave up "Muffins with Mom", chaperoned field trips, and innumerable other activities because I needed to work. Still, you always speak of me proudly and without any hint of resentment. You have grown into such talented, kind, and generous young men. I must have done something pretty amazing in a prior life to have been given the honor of being your mother in this one.

Alefiyah. I may be the older sister, but you have wisdom beyond your years. Thank you for being a daily example of the importance of living your dream. I so often get bogged down in the routine and responsibilities of daily life, but you see the big picture and live for it. Your commitment to "following your arrow" is an inspiration to me.

Drs. Raoul Wolf, Anita Gewurz, James Moy, Mary Kay Tobin, Byung Yu, and Giselle Mosnaim. Thank you for providing me such an excellent foundation in allergy and clinical immunology, and for teaching me to balance a commitment to evidence-based medicine with the ability to think outside of the box.

The hundreds of pioneers of modern food allergen desensitization, both in academia and in private practice. Thank you for designing, implementing, interpreting, and freely sharing your work with the world. Medicine only improves when we continue to innovate, integrate, and build upon existing knowledge. Thank you for laying the foundation.

Dr. Richard Wasserman. Thank you for sharing your experience and knowledge with a young and earnest colleague. Thank you for keeping a laser-focus on patient welfare, and for not being dissuaded by the naysayers. You have truly blazed a trail in our specialty, and your mentorship has been invaluable, not only to me, but also to hundreds of other allergists.

Drs. Douglas Jones and Hugh Windom. You recognized the need for a physician-led organization (Food Allergy Support Team) to ensure that those of us in the trenches had a powerful voice in shaping the future of food allergen desensitization for our patients. Thank you for trusting me to play a role in this endeavor. You also saw the wisdom of creating a mechanism for collecting valuable data from private OIT practices and pooling it to advance patient safety. Thank you for working so hard to make the OIT registry a reality.

All my allergist colleagues performing food allergen desensitization in academic and private practice. Thank you for your commitment to collaboration and ongoing improvement. I am so honored to be a part of this community of physicians that changes lives every day.

Bonnie Punter. My right-hand woman. Thank you for keeping Kaneland Allergy and Asthma Center humming, and for giving 110 percent every day. You are all heart, and I am blessed to have you in my circle.

Ankita Shah. Thank you for the thoughtful and compassionate care you provide to our patients, and for being an all-around lovely person to work with. It is truly a pleasure to collaborate with such a kind and intelligent colleague each day.

Ashley Wixom, Amy Brooks, Kristina Lex, Tracy Strasser.

Thank you all for the dedication you have shown in providing excellent care to every patient who passes through our doors. It takes special people to work in a small medical practice like ours, and I am so proud of the role each of you has played in our work.

To all the students and trainees who have passed through my office. Thank you for choosing Kaneland Allergy and Asthma Center to expand your education in allergy and immunology. Teaching helps me become a better educator and physician. I hope what you have learned with me helps shape your view of what patient-centered care can be.

Liseetsa Mann. You weren't content to save only your own child. You set out to save a generation. You have created a vibrant community of patients, families, and healthcare professionals who share your passion for improving awareness of and access to food desensitization therapy. Thank you for your devoted work and your unfailing support. #OITworks

Gail Reynolds. You could have sailed off into the sunset, but instead you worked tirelessly to create an enduring online resource to connect patients with OIT allergists. What an incredible effort.

Women Physician Writers. Your encouragement and advice kept me going when I felt overwhelmed. I'm so grateful for a community of physician writers with whom to share trials and triumphs.

Food Allergy Physician Moms. Thank you for sharing your insights into parenting children with food allergies, from the perspective of both mother and physician. It helped me focus this book on the topics that matter most.

Dawn Eby and Nadia Khambati. Thank you for volunteering your time and expertise to the Kaneland Food Allergy Foundation. We are so thankful to have you on board to help fulfill our mission.

Pete Lewis. Thank you for your accounting expertise and assistance in establishing the Kaneland Food Allergy Foundation.

Kenneth Gay and BeQRious. Thank you for creating such dynamic QR codes to link to our video content. Beqrioustracker.com: 'Making QR Codes That Help Your Business Grow.'

Rahil Calcuttawala and Rakimagery. Thank you for your assistance in creating our educational videos.

Advocate Sherman Hospital. Thank you for supporting your staff physicians in their endeavors, and for the use of your video and audio equipment.

Tucker Max. My friend of more than twenty years. Thank you for creating Scribe to help give voice to the stories we hold in our hearts and minds.

My excellent publishing team at Scribe: Emily Gindlesparger, Claire Winters, Jessica Burdg, Sheila Trask. Thank you for lending your talents to this project. Throughout the process, I was impressed with your professionalism, responsiveness, and attention to detail. The "A-Team," indeed.

My tribe. How do I even begin to explain what your support means to me? I think Jennifer Pastiloff said it best: "You know, the ones that make you feel the most YOU. The ones that lift you up and help you remember who you really are. The ones that remind you that a blip in the road is just that, a blip, and not to mistake it for an earthquake, and even it were to be an earthquake, they'd be there with the Earthquake Emergency Supply Kit. They are the ones that, when you walk out of a room, they make you feel like a better person than when you walked in. They are the ones that, even if you don't see them face to face as often as you'd like, you see them heart to heart."

My dear patients. There would be no book if not for your courage in facing the unknown and taking a chance to achieve the limitless future you deserve. You are my heroes.

Courage is the most important of all the virtues, because without courage you can't practice any other virtue consistently. You can practice any virtue erratically, but nothing consistently without courage.

—MAYA ANGELOU

From the bottom of my heart, thank you all.

ABOUT THE AUTHOR

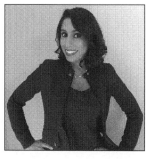

DR. SAKINA SHIKARI BAJOWALA is a board-certified adult and pediatric allergist and immunologist with a passion for patient education and advocacy. In her private allergy practice, she helps her young patients overcome food allergies through precision-focused sublingual and oral immunotherapy.

As an allergy sufferer herself and a mother to allergic children, Dr. Bajowala is known for her compassionate bedside manner and individualized treatment plans that draw from a variety of medical disciplines. She believes in educating and empowering patients to optimize health by teaching them to understand how their bodies work. Visit SakinaBajowala.com.

Made in the USA
Monee, IL
09 February 2020